D1824387

Healthy Eating for Healthy Living

A Complete guide to zero sugar diet for beginners

By Christina J Evans

Table of Contents

Just for You

A free gift to our readers

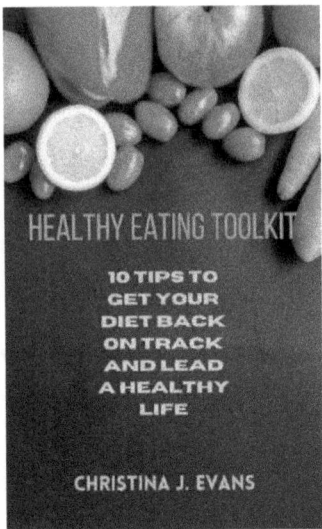

Click here

http://christinajevans.com/healthy-eating.pdf

Joining the HL Community

Looking to build your healthy eating lifestyle? If so, then check out the Healthy Living (HL) Community here:

www.facebook.com/groups/1004091000384321/

Introduction

*I*t was a normal Friday. At least I thought so. *My youngest daughter, Evie, had a bake sale at school so I was up to my arms in cookie dough and muffin batter the previous day. I have to say I was happy with the results. So much so, that I didn't mind sampling 'a few'.*

The following day, I brought my daughter to school, and just when we were about to enter, she turned around, reached for the bag of baked goodies, looked up to me, and said "It's ok mommy. You don't have to go with me." I was surprised but I let her go, thinking she was probably trying to be a 'big girl'.

At the end of the school day, I was outside waiting for her when one of the other moms came up to me and said "Hey, you feeling better now?" Seeing my confused look, she said, "Evie said you were not feeling well and asked one of the other moms to help her with the bake sale." Somehow, I managed a "Yes, I feel better now" - just at the exact time I was feeling worse.

When I tucked my little girl that night I asked her as casually as I can "Why didn't you want mommy to help you out today?"

She looked at me and said "I don't like it when the other kids call you the 'black tent lady'. You know, because you only wear big, black clothes all the time." Oh. "And you probably couldn't help anyway." Oh? "We had to go set up outside and do A LOT of stuff and the other mommies are faster moving around, and going up and down the stairs. You're too fat to do that." And then she turned around and pretended to sleep.

And just like that – my heart broke into a thousand pieces.

That was the turning point for me.

FOR YOU – I'm sure you've had your own turning point as well.

- It can be seeing yourself in a photo and then suddenly being shocked at how 'big' you've become.
- It can be that judgmental look that complete strangers give you as they stare at your size. (It's worse when they do that at the grocery store or while you're dining in a restaurant.)
- It can be a friend, colleague, or family member 'innocently' making fun of your weight.
- It can be people always asking if you're pregnant.

- It can be the saleslady telling you that you should really try the dress you're holding in a bigger size.
- Worse still... depression may be hitting you or a serious health issue has come up that's completely negatively impacting your way of life. (You may even think – what life?)

I know all this because **I've been in your shoes**. In fact, ALL of the items above happened to me at one point or the other.

I wish I could tell you that from my turning point, all the excess pounds dropped easily and we lived happily ever after. But that was not the case. **I failed so many times.**

Over the next three (3) years, I would lose weight, gain weight... lose weight, gain weight... In the end, **I had put on MORE weight than when I started**. It was a very mentally draining and emotionally exhausting time. Every time I gained the weight back **I would sink into depression.**

The depression got so bad that at one point, **I started to become physically ill**. I would have panic attacks while driving, blinding migraines that prevented sleep, and during one beach vacation – yes, I was wearing something big and black to cover up myself again – **I had a heart attack**. My doctor said that I either had to be on medication for the rest of my life or lose weight.

By this time, I just wanted to throw my hands in the air. The only thing that stopped me from completely giving up was this **– I couldn't find the words to tell my daughter 'yes, mommy's a failure'**.

So for the nth time, **I tried again.**

And **THIS time, everything fell into place. I lost the weight - and successfully kept it off - for 10 years now.** And I couldn't be happier with my life!

- Imagine waking up wide-eyed, alert, and full of energy.
- Think of all the health issues – shortness of breath, all-day tiredness, heart problems, diabetes, joint pain, high cholesterol, etc. – that can be REVERSED.
- Visualize cutting your food budget by almost 50%(!) not by eating less, but by eating right.
- Look years younger as you see your hair, skin and overall appearance dramatically improve.
-

- Wear anything you want! Picture a wardrobe that's not 'all black and baggy' but made up of various styles, cuts, and colors you can wear confidently.

And perhaps best of all – imagine looking in the mirror and loving who and what you see.

Now, I don't think there's a woman alive out there who doesn't want at least one of the things I listed above, so let me tell you exactly what's going to happen.

I'm going to hold your hand and give you my step-by-step tested blueprint on how to cut sugar from your life so that you can quickly and successfully lose weight, and not gain a single pound back.

You see, I know what you're going through because believe me, **I've been there**. I've gone through so many 'fad diets' that I almost completely wrecked my health and my body.

So when I opened my eyes and understood that **we were being fed LIE after LIE after LIE about how to lose weight**, uncovering the TRUTH became my goal.

Instead of just believing in whatever an 'overnight guru' was talking about, I buried myself in RESEARCH. Science became my friend. Licensed doctors specializing in female weight loss became my allies. This is why through the next pages you will see me frequently refer to published data and studies. **There is no hype here. Just truths.**

When I had collected enough knowledge, I created a **zero sugar weight loss plan** for myself. And I am not kidding when I tell you that **the pounds just started to melt away**.

All the hardship, all the illness, all the heartaches, all the disappointments – they disappeared as my excess weight melted away.

Soon enough, EVERY SINGLE PERSON I came into contact with would remark about my amazing transformation. Some would just ask how I did it, but many more would beg me to create a zero sugar weight loss plan for them too!

And I could never say no. How can I when I've been living under the shadow of obesity too for many years? And when you start to uncover what works, you always say to yourself – *if only someone told me the right way to successfully lose weight, and keep it off.*

Well then, **let me be that SOMEONE.**

If you're ready to drop the weight and change your life – **turn the page** and keep reading.

To your healthy living,

Christina J. Evans
Female Body Fat Expert | Healthy Living Advocate

Chapter 1

Healthy Eating Guidelines

QUALITY OF LIFE. Many eBooks on healthy eating focus on weight loss and looking good. There is, of course, absolutely nothing wrong with the physical or aesthetic consequences of eating healthy. However, you should also keep in mind that with healthy eating you also achieve BETTER QUALITY OF LIFE.

Think about **living WITHOUT suffering from health- and weight-related diseases** such as diabetes, coronary heart disease, high cholesterol, high blood pressure, and so on.

Think about the **MENTAL AND EMOTIONAL STABILITY** that you will achieve if you NOURISH your body with good, quality food rather than just 'filling it'.

WHAT is Healthy Eating?

Healthy eating is eating REAL FOOD. It is ensuring that you are feeding your body with nutritious food and drinks to help it function at its best. It also means following a healthy eating pattern and consuming the right amount of healthy calories for your body.

WHY Should You Eat Healthily?

There are so many reasons to live a healthy life. And here are some of those reasons.

> ➤ Improve HEART health.
>
> Did you know that **heart disease is the primary cause of death for adults in the US?[1]** That sounds a bit grim but here's the good news – up to 80% of premature heart disease and stroke occurrences are preventable IF you adopt a healthy living lifestyle!
>
> A zero sugar diet automatically helps to lower blood pressure and keep your heart healthy. So you're on the right track .

> ➤ Lower your cancer risk.
>
> Eating healthy, good-quality food items means you're also eating food rich in antioxidants, substances that can prevent or slow damage to cells caused by free radicals. This in turn reduces your chance of contracting serious illnesses such as cancer.

Some studies have also found that a diet high in fruits lowered the risk of upper gastrointestinal tract cancers.

> **Improve GUT health.**
>
Our bodies serve as a host to a myriad of bacteria. This is a fact. The key is to keep a healthy balance between good and bad bacteria. If bad bacteria start to thrive in our bodies, our immune system weakens making it vulnerable to various diseases.

A diet low in fiber and high in sugar and fat promotes the growth of harmful bacteria. So switching to a zero sugar diet is definitely beneficial for your gut health.

> **Strengthen your bones and teeth.**
>
One of the things that people don't realize is that by NOT eating healthy food, your body loses out on much-needed nutrients. For instance, calcium and magnesium are important for strong bones and teeth. You simply cannot squeeze these nutrients out of a *hotdog*.

> **Improve brain function.**
>
Research shows that certain nutrients and foods improve brain function and protect against cognitive decline and dementia. A low carbohydrate, zero sugar diet rich in vitamins, omega-3 fatty acids, flavonoids and polyphenols, and fish were in particular seen as great for improving brain health.

> **Sleep better.**
>
Do you sleep well? It sounds like an easy enough question, but did you know that 62% of adults around the world claim that they don't sleep as well as they would

like.[2] If you don't get good quality sleep, instead of feeling rejuvenated the next day, you feel sleepy, foggy, and groggy. And this leads to bad eating choices, which in turn can lead to weight gain. How?

Some studies have shown that sleep deprivation lowers *leptin* (the hormone that tells your brain you're full) and increases *ghrelin* (the hormone that tells your brain you're hungry).[3]

So what you should keep in mind here is that one completely affects the other. If you don't sleep well, it's highly possible you'll eat more and make bad eating choices the next day (weight gain). But if you DO eat well, you increase your chances of sleeping well. So win-win!

> BE HAPPY.

We are what we eat. Studies show a direct link between what we eat and our mood. In fact, a 2016 study discovered that a **diet with a high glycemic load may cause symptoms of depression and fatigue.**[4]

NOTE:

You've probably heard of the glycemic index (GI). This indicates how fast 50g of carbs in a particular food item raises our blood glucose levels.

The glycemic load (GL), on the other hand, considers GI values <u>and</u> the total amount of carbohydrates in a standard food serving. As such, it indicates a food item's glycemic and insulin response.

See also <u>Appendix A</u> for a list of common grocery items and their glycemic load.

In another study, it was learned that a diet rich in vitamins and minerals is linked to a lower risk for mental health disorders including anxiety, depression, and attention-deficit hyperactivity disorder (ADHD).[5]

And let's face it - success at any endeavor makes one happy! Doing a zero sugar diet and succeeding at your weight and health goals are all excellent reasons to be happy.

> LOSE WEIGHT!

Excess weight increases your risk for chronic diseases. Luckily, a healthy eating lifestyle automatically promotes weight loss!

By simply focusing on the RIGHT FOOD to eat, you inevitably lower your calorie consumption. So, if you're worried about 'calorie counting', don't be.

Eat well and eat right and dropping the pounds will follow.

7 Tips to Increase Your Chances of Healthy Eating Success

In Chapter 7, you'll get a detailed zero sugar diet plan. But to give you the best chance of success, I suggest that you first do the following so that you're in the RIGHT

ENVIRONMENT to succeed with your healthy eating, healthy living plan.

1. **Start SLOW.**

   Change is difficult. Many people who want to change their eating lifestyles do so with the best intentions. However, taking on too much too soon is detrimental to success.

   Think of it this way – **success builds on success**.

   You may start slow, but as the days progress you will notice small changes. For example, you may start to notice that you breathe easier, or that you have a bit more energy in the mornings, you may even start to notice some weight loss. Take each achievement and build upon it.

On the other hand, if you make too many life changes at once, you may not be able to keep up with all of them. Things may begin to feel too difficult, making you give up and stop any progress.

2.   **Switch to smaller plates.**
Did you know that a bigger plate can make you eat more?[6] This is because our eyes like to see a full plate – no matter what its size. The great thing about switching to smaller plates is that you trick your brain and your stomach to eat less without even noticing!

If you don't want to switch to smaller plates completely then switch what you PUT on your plates. For example, put healthier food items on your normal-sized plate, and less healthy ones on a smaller plate.

3.   **Keep a food journal.**
Many dieters underestimate the power of keeping a food journal. In one study, it was found that people who kept a food diary six days a week lost about twice as much weight![7] Here are some of the reasons why keeping a food diary works.

- **You become mindful of WHAT you eat.**
    Mindless eating or distracted eating is when a person is completely unaware of what or how much food (and drink!) he or she is consuming. This is why so many dieters THINK they're eating less, but in reality, they're not eating less at all. In fact, they may be eating MORE. Why? Many people who go on a weight loss program overestimate the energy they burn and underestimate the calories they consume.

    However, if you keep a food journal then you know exactly WHAT you've eaten and HOW MUCH you've consumed. But this is only half the equation. Once you have this knowledge then *healthy adjustments* need to kick in.

    For example, say you noticed you eat two (2) chocolate chip cookies every afternoon with your coffee. The average chocolate chip cookie contains approximately 200 calories. So now you know you consume 400 calories every afternoon just on two cookies!

    Healthy adjustment #1 -> consume only one cookie for a week
    Healthy adjustment #2 -> consume a different, healthier cookie for a week
    Healthy adjustment #3 -> substitute fruit for the cookie

Your 'healthy adjustments' are all up to you. The most important thing is that you apply them. If you can, go 'cold turkey' and simply eliminate eating

cookies with your mid-afternoon coffee. The most important thing is this: make a change that supports your new healthy eating ways.

- **You can keep track of any food allergies, issues, and sensitivities.**
  Keeping a food diary also helps you narrow down which food items may be causing problems such as headaches, bloating, indigestion, and others. For instance, she never really noticed it but after keeping a food journal a friend of mine noticed that chips (her weekend indulgence), and broccoli (one of her favorite healthy foods) were causing her bloating and flatulence! You can imagine how fast she got rid of those food items on her diet.

- **You can uncover unhealthy food triggers.**
  Are you a stress eater? An emotional eater? A habitual eater?

Stress eaters, as the name suggests, are those who eat when they feel anxious or pressured. An emotional eater usually uses food to comfort themselves such as when feeling lonely, depressed, or bored. A habitual eater is someone who eats simply out of routine. For instance, many people tend to bring out the 'munchies' when watching TV after dinner. You're not necessarily hungry; you're just used to eating something while in front of the TV.

Discover your trigger for unhealthy eating, and you'll find a way to 'de-activate' your eating response.

For example, a friend of mine noticed that one of her food triggers is when she dropped off her son at her ex-husband's place for the weekend. She would come back home and start looking for things to eat. (Her food journal showed a long list of food items every other Friday night.)

So to STOP this eating response, she started planning activities after dropping her son off. She visited a local swimming club and has been swimming every Friday night since then.

How to start a food journal.

A lot of people don't start a food journal because they overthink it! So just start. Don't worry about fancy pens, notebooks, and paper. Grab anything you can use. Although you can also just use your mobile device, writing them down is better.

Also, keeping a food diary is a habit you need to develop. So don't be discouraged if you fail to log something or skip a day or two. Focus instead

on trying to develop a routine. Log items (what you eat AND drink) as soon as they pass your lips.

Log how you feel too after consuming something. For instance, after a specific meal or food item, do you feel good or stuffed? Energetic or sluggish? Take note and adjust accordingly.

BE HONEST. No one else is going to benefit from your food journal except you. So, there's no point in fibbing the details. By knowing and accepting what you've done, only then can you make positive changes.

4. **Acquire a support system.**
When embarking on a weight loss program, you may want to start 'quietly'. However, having a support system can dramatically increase your chances of long-term weight loss success. And I'm not just talking about friends and family members. Of course, if they support you, great! But your weight loss support system can come from other corners too.

Look around you. Do you have friends or colleagues interested in losing weight too? If so, talk to these people. Perhaps you can find a co-worker with whom you can have 'walk dates' after lunch or a friend with whom you can plan healthy cooking weekends.

Join your local gym. It's already filled with people concerned about healthy living, so you just might find your new fitness buddy there.

Consider online weight loss groups or forums too. There are A LOT of online groups dedicated to healthy eating and healthy living, and perhaps you'll find the support and help you need there.

You are making a huge, positive life change right now. And you don't need to do it alone.

Look around. Don't be scared. Ask for help.

You just might be surprised at how much your circle can GROW by simply reaching out.

5. **Minimize distractions.**

Often, life gets in the way of weight loss plans. You know how it is. A friend calls for a lunch date at a restaurant with too many high-sugar, high-calorie choices.

Work deadlines mean working late (again?) and so you're 'forced' to order in food. There are many ways your best-laid healthy eating plans can be sabotaged.

However, you know all of this already, which means you can plan ahead and be ready for such distractions. Here are some tips.

- **Meal prep during the weekend.** You know that there will be times when you simply don't have enough time to cook a healthy meal. Fine. You know this. Accept it. Now, what are you going to do about it? You meal prep. Make a shortlist of quick and healthy meals you can cook or prep over the weekend, portion these out, and put them in your freezer. This way, you'll have a ready supply of healthy meals within arm's reach.

    And don't think healthy meals are bland or boring! Are chicken nuggets boring?!? (Click here for healthy, REAL Chicken Nuggets recipe.)

- **STOP checking your mobile phone and/or computer first thing in the morning.** Focus first on having a HEALTHY breakfast, and perhaps even getting a short workout done in the morning before you put your mind on work mode.

- **Learn to say NO.** Saying no to someone or something is not being mean or selfish. It's simply you loving and prioritizing enough to focus on your health and fitness. Remember, you're supposed to live YOUR life, not someone else's. So do things that benefit YOU.

6. **Think of NON-FOOD related rewards.**

An eating lifestyle high in sugar conditions the brain to seek food as a reward. So before you embark on your zero sugar diet, have a go-to list of non-food related rewards.

For example, instead of a 'cheat day', reward yourself with a 'spa day' when you reach a certain weight milestone.

Here are other non-food related ideas to treat yourself.

1) Go for a new haircut.
2) Buy a new dress.
3) Buy/read a book.
4) **Schedule a Netflix 'marathon'.**
5) Book a massage.
6) Drive somewhere.
7) Book a facial.
8) Call someone and schedule an impromptu dinner or movie date (or both!).
9) Purchase a cooking gadget or utensil that supports your new zero sugar, low carbohydrate lifestyle (e.g., juicer, steamer, etc.)
10) Get new sports clothes/gear.
11) Take a day off.
12) Buy yourself some flowers.

7.   KEEP AN OPEN MIND!

Lastly, and perhaps the best tip of all – **keep an open mind. Don't limit yourself.**

Don't disregard something just because it's new or you're not used to it.

In fact, many people new to the healthy eating for healthy living movement never thought they would end up loving something they've never tried before such as meal prepping or even cooking in general.

Remember, just because you've never tried it before, doesn't mean you can't or won't like it.

Chapter 2
The ZERO SUGAR Diet and How It Works

What's Wrong with Sugar?

Sugar is naturally present in small quantities in vegetables, fruits, grains, and dairy. Eating whole foods that contain **NATURAL SUGAR** is okay because, in addition to sugar, real food is also high in fiber, essential minerals, antioxidants, protein, calcium, and a host of other good things that your body needs to function well.

And since our bodies digest real food slowly, the naturally occurring sugar in them provides a steady flow of energy into our bodies' cells. (No sugar rush!)

The problem starts when we eat too much **ADDED SUGAR**. This is the sugar that food **manufacturers add to their products to boost flavor, texture, and extend**

shelf life.

Keep in mind that **ADDED SUGARS do not provide any nutritional value or benefit whatsoever.** What do they add? **EMPTY CALORIES**, which lead to weight gain and illness.

Here are some quick ADDED SUGAR facts for you:

- Most added sugar comes from prepared and processed foods.

- Soft drinks and breakfast cereals are the grocery staples that contain the most added sugars.

- The average soft drink can contain 150 calories, most of which come from high-fructose corn syrup. This is roughly the equivalent of 10 teaspoons of table sugar!

High fructose corn syrup, derived from *corn starch*, is way cheaper and sweeter than normal sugar. It's absorbed by the body faster (sugar rush!), and is linked to insulin resistance, obesity, Type 2 diabetes, and high blood pressure.

- The American Heart Association recommends added sugar consumption to be no more than 100 calories per day for women (6 teaspoons or 24 grams of sugar), and no more than 150 calories per day for men (9 teaspoons or 36 grams).[8] However, most Americans consume more than 19 teaspoons of added sugar (290 calories) per day!

HOT TIP: When buying something, quickly go over the nutritional label of the food item. If 'sugar' is listed as the first or second ingredient, then skip that product as you're basically just adding calories to your diet.

See also **Appendix B** for a list of the most common names for sugar.

Ok, so now you know that ADDED SUGAR is all around you and that's one of the reasons why you consume so much of it. Basically, you UNKNOWINGLY consume a lot of added sugar.

Another reason we consume so much added sugar is that research has shown that it's biologically addicting.[9]

Sugar causes *dopamine* to be released in the reward center of the brain. This response is similar to what addictive drugs do. If you consume a lot of sugar, you're reinforcing this 'reward' pattern, making it difficult to break such a habit.

Also ever wondered why you get such a 'rush' after eating candy, a cookie, or a piece of chocolate cake? This is because the added sugar in these food items quickly turns into glucose in your bloodstream, resulting in a 'sugar high'. However, the 'high' fizzles out fast and now you experience a sudden drop in energy. What do you do?

You look for more sweets to regain that 'sugar high'. So what you're really just doing is reinforcing a bad eating habit that's making you fat and unhealthy.

By the way, **sugar is NOT all about sweets**. Flour-based foods such as your favorite baked goods (donuts, pies, cake, white bread, pasta, etc.) are complex carbs that the body breaks down into simple sugars.

And sugar can 'hide' too. They may not taste sweet but items like ketchup, barbecue sauce, pasta sauce, flavored coffees, and reduced-fat salad dressings, can be high in sugar.

With all of the above, you're probably thinking...

Am I doomed to consume sugar? **No, you're not.**
Don't I have a choice? **Yes, you do.**
Can't I make a change? **Yes, you can!**

Following a zero sugar diet can retrain your taste buds so that you break that bad sugar habit! And in the process, I promise that you will live your best life yet.

Why Eliminate Added Sugar?

Oh boy, where do we start? Following are some of the known dangers of consuming too much added sugar.

Obesity

Studies show that those who follow **diets high in added sugar are more likely to develop obesity.**[10]

Studies show that high-sugar, high-carb diets lead to an unhealthy gut, which is one of the reasons for the development of obesity.

Also, unlike previous years, today's diet includes a lot of soda consumption. These drinks are high in sugar, which leads to a high-calorie intake. This doesn't only lead to weight gain, but to a decrease in the consumption of other important nutrients too!

Cancer

Research on lab rats found that a high-sugar diet may increase the development of breast cancer.

In another study involving more than 35,000 women, it was found that a high-sugar eating lifestyle nearly had twice the risk of developing colon cancer, compared to subjects who followed a diet with less added sugar.

The theory is that high (added) sugar intake leads to inflammation. And in the long-term, this sugar-caused inflammation damages the body's cells and its innate ability to fight off diseases.

Insulin Resistance

Studies show that when you consume more added sugar than you should, excess glucose is produced in the body. When this happens, **insulin resistance** occurs, which can lead to the development of **prediabetes**, and eventually **Type 2 diabetes**.

High insulin levels from consuming too much sugar are also believed to increase one's risk of developing cancer.

Oral Health

A **high sugar diet is also linked to bad oral health**[11] such as oral infections and ulcers, tooth decay, halitosis (bad breath), oral thrush, gum disease, and others.

Fatigue, stress and anxiety, joint pain, skin problems, acid reflux, and irritable bowel syndrome are also all linked to a high sugar diet.

As you can see, a high-sugar diet can wreak havoc on your health. If you adopt a zero sugar diet, you're not just addressing one health issue. You are managing and preventing A LOT of potential health problems.

What is the ZERO SUGAR diet?

In a nutshell, a zero sugar diet is an eating lifestyle wherein the focus is on consuming nutritious high-fiber foods, such as whole grains, fruits, vegetables, and nuts, as well as lean protein.

A sugar-free diet aims to 'flush out' sugar and its negative effects on your body completely. It will reset your brain back to the state when it was not craving sugar as much as you do now, breaking your body's dependence on it.

A zero sugar lifestyle also means you'll be FREE from the roller coaster sugar highs and lows that have a negative effect on your daily energy, mood, and waistline.

The Link Between Sugar and Carbs

As you go on a zero sugar eating lifestyle, you'll find that you automatically adopt a low carbohydrate diet as well. This is because carbs and sugar are linked to each other.

For starters, **sugars, starches, and fiber are carbohydrates**.

Complex Carbohydrates

Complex carbs contain naturally-occurring sugars that are harder to break down (in the body) and thus take longer to digest. And as mentioned above, a STEADY flow of sugar prevents sugar highs and crashes and is thus beneficial to weight loss and overall health.

Complex carbs also have prebiotic properties that support the growth of good bacteria in the gut. In addition, they are high in fiber and nutrients, which help to make us feel fuller for longer periods of time.

Simple Carbohydrates

Simple carbs are fast-digesting sugars. They can be present in complex carbohydrates, but they are mostly found in BIG quantities in processed foods. Processed foods often include refined sugars that are extracted and purified from plants, like sugar beets, sugar cane, and corn.

Simple carbs are NOT nutritious. And since they break down easily in the body, you don't feel full for longer. As a result, you reach out for these types of foods (again!) more easily. This, of course, leads to an excessive intake of calories.

Our body needs complex carbohydrates in order to function. The glucose they provide is the main fuel source for the brain and it's needed for proper muscle function. We don't need simple carbohydrates as they have little to no nutritional value. So, given the above, the best way to go low carbohydrate is to stick to complex carbs and get rid of simple carbs (or at the very least, limit your consumption of it).

The Effects of Going 'Low Carb' on Your Body

There are three macronutrients found in food.

1. **Carbohydrates** (4 kcal/gm)
2. **Fat** (9 kcal/gm)
3. **Protein** (4 kcal/gm)

As such, studies have defined 'low carbohydrate' as a percent of daily macronutrient intake or total daily carbohydrate load.[12] In particular:

- Very low carbohydrate (< 10% carbohydrates) or 20-50 gm/day
- **low carbohydrate (<26% carbohydrates) or less than < 130 gm/day**
- Moderate carbohydrate (26%-44%)
- High carbohydrate (45% or greater)

When you begin a low carbohydrate diet, your body will of course notice something different. It will be on a search for more sugar to burn for fuel.

Without getting the sugar it needs from food, your blood sugar levels will lower and your cortisol levels will rise. Cortisol is a hormone released by your adrenal glands to confirm

you have enough energy to survive.

When your blood sugar levels are low, your brain sends a signal to your adrenal glands

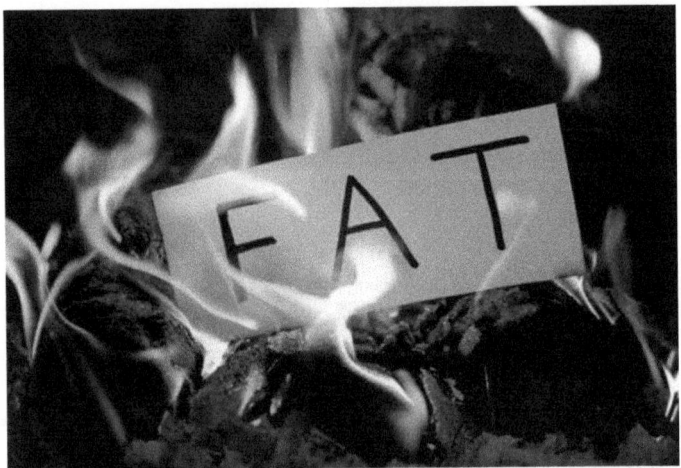

to release cortisol. The cortisol then starts a process called *gluconeogenesis*, which tells your body to convert protein and fat into sugar.

This is the stage low carbohydrate dieters want –> when the body starts to adapt by burning fat for fuel instead of protein. This is called ketosis.

Basically, ketosis is the body's method of ensuring you don't burn away muscle mass and glycogen during times of carbohydrate and/or protein restriction.

However, note that ketosis is NOT an overnight event. It can take a few days before your body enters into *ketosis*, which may leave you stressed, fatigued, and weak.

Now, you may be thinking... is it worth it?

To burn fat for fuel, should you go low on carbohydrates and put your body through all this 'stress'? Studies think so. One study showed that the increase in cortisol levels on a low carbohydrate diet was trivial when compared to the cortisol levels of people on moderate and high-carb diets.

What other results can you expect from a low carbohydrate diet?

> **You'll feel less hungry.**
> What makes you feel full? What satiates hunger?

Nutrients - fiber, protein, and healthy fats – make you feel full. Empty calories (from simple carbs and added sugars) do not satisfy hunger. So a low carbohydrate diet

➢ **You'll lose belly fat.**

When you go low carbohydrate, your food choices tend to go high fiber. And that's a great thing! Most Americans on average consume only 15 grams of fiber daily, against the 19-38 grams per day recommended by the Institute of Medicine.[13]

What's the connection? Fiber is needed by our healthy gut microbes. A diet rich in simple carbs and sugar promotes the growth of bad gut bacteria, which in turn promotes consistent bloating.

➢ **You'll build muscle.**

Simple carbohydrates lack protein, the building blocks of muscle. By filling your body with protein and other nutrients, you're giving your muscles what it needs to develop without having to find additional calories. Also, an overweight body *covers* muscles with fat. But since you're burning fat in a low carbohydrate diet, your muscles will now have a chance to show. (Hello, toned body!)

➢ **You'll feel more energized.**

Since you're consuming food that provides body fuel for longer periods of time, you'll have a steady - and non-fluctuating! - source of energy. Ever wondered why healthy people don't seem to ever go 'low bat'? This is the reason.

> ➢ **And of course, you'll lose weight!**
>
>   If you follow a low carbohydrate diet well, your body will enter ketosis and burn stored fat. This is why low carbohydrate diets are seen as a means for rapid weight loss!

However, in the interest of completeness, note that going low on carbohydrates can also have some less-than-appealing side effects.

You see, ketosis is NOT an overnight event. It can take a few days before your body enters into ketosis, which can result in the following side effects.

- Headache/migraines
- Bad breath (halitosis)
- Weakness
- Fatigue
- Constipation or diarrhea
- Hair loss

Although some may experience the above negative side effects, many people on a low carbohydrate diet do not report them at all.

To be on the safe side, always consult a physician before embarking on any new dietary change. And be vigilant about your own body! Monitor how your body is reacting to changes, and react accordingly.

Low Carbohydrate Diets and Hydration

When your carbohydrate intake is very low, the insulin levels in your body go low too. And when insulin is low, your liver starts to burn fat and make ketones (*ketosis*). However, low insulin levels have other effects. Low insulin also results in water, sodium, and potassium loss through urine.[14] This means that a very low carbohydrate diet increases your body's needs for both fluids and electrolytes.

This is why some people tend to suffer from dehydration at the start of a very low carbohydrate diet. The lack of fluids results in cramps, fatigue, and headaches... also known as the *keto flu*.

Now you may think that to battle keto flu, you should simply drink A LOT of water. Not quite.

Remember, you're losing water AND electrolytes. If you drink too much water, you run the risk of diluting blood sodium levels and thus boost the risk of *hyponatremia* (low sodium condition state).

So how do you stay properly hydrated on a low carbohydrate diet? Researchers believe in the following principles:

1. **Drink water when thirsty.**

   Here's a tip: if you get tired of drinking plain water, then drink fruit-flavored water. But don't just use any fruit as they may have a high glycemic load. (You will just be reversing the effects of your ketosis if you drink sugar-heavy drinks, even if they are natural sugars.) Use berries or citrus peels to flavor your water.

2. **Consume enough electrolytes.**

   Consume fluid-balancing electrolytes (sodium and potassium) through food and supplements. This means you should **eat a lot of potassium-rich leafy greens** such as Swiss chard, beet greens, lima beans, acorn squash, spinach, pakchoi (bok choy), white button mushrooms, tomatoes, Brussel sprouts, broccoli, green peas, and fennel.

   You should also **add a bit more salt to your food than you would normally consume**. Salt your eggs, your rice, meat, etc. The recommended daily limit on salt intake is 2.3 grams per day. However, since you're trying to up your electrolytes, you can consume around 5 grams of sodium per day (about 2.5 teaspoons of salt).

You may also **consider taking a high-quality supplement** that contains plenty of sodium. Ideally, a supplement with at least 500 mg of sodium per serving.

There's another reason to ensure you're properly hydrated during a low carbohydrate diet – *keto breath.*

The ketones produced in your body during ketosis are released through your breath as acetone. Some people report a fruity or sweet breath scent. Others, however, liken the breath to rotten apples or nail polish remover. And if you don't hydrate well, you'll suffer from a dry mouth, which means there's not enough saliva to remove bacteria and food particles in your mouth. So - stay hydrated!

And since keto breath is not at all sexy, here are more tips to avoid it.

> ➢ Improve oral hygiene.
> In addition to brushing your teeth after each meal, consider the following oral hygiene practices too:

- **Floss away.** Flossing is a great way to get rid of food particles stuck between your teeth. You may already practice this before you sleep but consider doing it after every meal. You don't want those food particles to rot and cause even more unpleasant breath, do you?

- **Clean and scrape your tongue.** Consider buying a tongue scraper to rid your tongue of bacteria. One study found that tongue scraping twice a day for a week lowered the presence of *Mutans streptococci* and *Lactobacilli bacteria* in the mouth. These bacteria are credited to induce bad breath and tooth decay.[15]

- **Give 'oil pulling' a try.** Coconut oil is known for its antibacterial properties. To oil pull, swirl a small amount of coconut oil in your mouth and in between your teeth. This swishing 'pulls' unfriendly bacteria from your tongue, gums, cheek walls, etc., and gets eliminated when you spit.

> ➤   Drink LEMON water.

In addition to helping, you replenish your electrolytes, lemons also contain antibacterial properties. So, you get hydrated, and you rid your mouth of odor-causing bacteria.

> ➤   Try natural breath fresheners.

At the first sign of bad breath, you may want to turn to gum and fresh mints. Don't! These products are usually loaded with added sugars. Before you know it, you're out of ketosis faster than it took you to get to that state.

A better alternative is to turn to natural breath fresheners such as mint, sage, fennel seeds, parsley, cinnamon, clove, marjoram, and cardamom.

Don't want to chew the real thing? Look for all-natural extracts of these herbs and use them as a mouth spray.

Chapter 3
How to Break Away from Sugar

Food Habits to Break Away from Sugar for Life

Eat breakfast.

B reakfast is important. However, it's not the act of having it that makes you lose weight; it's the choices you make.

Many people think that by skipping breakfast, they reduce calorie consumption and thus lose weight. However, what happens in REAL LIFE is that by skipping breakfast, you lower your blood sugar levels so much so that by the time lunch comes around, you're so hungry that you make the WRONG food choices.

So don't skip breakfast. Instead, have a healthy zero sugar breakfast!
(Click here for low carb, zero sugar breakfast recipes.)

Sweeten foods naturally yourself.

So many food items have added sugars that it's now hard to determine what food tastes like naturally. So go back to basics and sweeten foods yourself. This means mostly using fruit as your sweetener. Stevia, a plant-based natural sweetener may also be used. However, apart from these, stay away from other sugar substitutes. This is because some sugar substitutes mess with your metabolism and even induce hunger.

Also, slowly lessen the amount of natural sweetener you use. For instance, if you use three (3) teaspoons of stevia for your morning steel-cut oatmeal, lower this to two (2) teaspoons after a week.

Schedule your meals.

It's all about balance and trying to maintain your blood sugar levels at a stable, non-roller-coaster pace. To achieve this, you need to evenly space out and schedule your meals during the day. The general rule is to eat a healthy meal every three to four hours. Of course, you may not always be able to keep to a tight schedule. As such, always keep healthy snacks such as cut vegetables, dried fruit, and raw nuts and seeds with you.

Meticulously plan your meals.

Scheduling your meals will not give you an ounce of benefit if you're not eating the right foods so plan exactly what you should be eating in advance. Meal prepping is crucial here so that you're not tempted to choose something else. Also, ensure that there's a protein in each meal.

Tip: Don't know how to plan your meals, follow my detailed 7-Day Zero-Sugar Diet Eating Plan.

Learn appropriate serving sizes.

Quick! What does a single serving of grilled chicken look like? It's ok if you don't know, A LOT of people don't. However, the fact remains that we unconsciously overeat because we're not aware of proper serving sizes.

So here's a breakdown of common food items and their recommended single-serving sizes.

- **Grains**

1 slice (40g) of bread

½ medium (40g) roll or flatbread

½ cup (75-120g) cooked rice, pasta, noodles, barley, buckwheat, semolina, polenta, bulgur, or quinoa

½ cup (120g) cooked porridge

2/3 cup (30g) wheat cereal flakes

¼ cup (30g) muesli

3 (35g) crispbreads

1 (60g) crumpet

1 small (35g) English muffin or scone

- **Vegetables**

½ cup cooked vegetables

½ cup cooked dried or canned beans

1 cup green leafy or raw salad vegetables

½ cup sweet corn

½ medium sweet potato

1 medium tomato

- **Fruits**

1 medium apple, banana, orange, or pear

2 small apricots, kiwi fruits, or plums

1 cup diced or canned fruit (no added sugar)

- **Protein foods (meat, poultry, fish, dry beans, and nuts)**

65g cooked lean red meat (about 90-100g raw)

80g cooked lean poultry (about 100g raw)

100g cooked fish fillet (about 115g raw, or one small can of fish)

2 large (120g) eggs

1 cup (150g) cooked or canned legumes or beans (e.g., lentils, chickpeas, split peas, etc.)

170g tofu

30g nuts or seeds

- **Dairy foods (milk, yogurt, and cheese)**

1 cup (250ml) fresh milk or buttermilk

2 slices (40g) hard cheese

½ cup (120g) ricotta cheese

¾ cup (200g) yogurt

1 cup (250ml) soy, rice, or other cereal drink

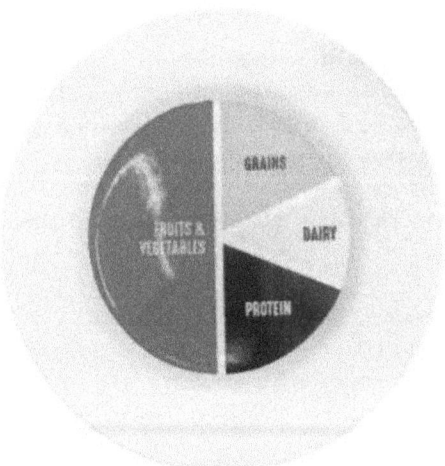

When you're at home, it's easy to keep track of the above. However, when eating out or at someone else's place, be guided visually by the following.

- One cup of raw leafy vegetables or a baked sweet potato should be around the size of a small fist.
- Three ounces of cooked poultry or lean meat should be around the size of a deck of cards.
- A teaspoon of soft margarine is about the size of a single die.
- An ounce and a half of fat-free or low-fat cheese are about the size of four stacked dice pieces.

Go for portion control.

Now that you know what a SINGLE serving of common food items is, how do you teach yourself not to go for more?

For starters, consider switching to a divided plate at home at the start of your weight loss journey.

This is just so you can get used to appropriate serving sizes. Soon enough, you'll find out that serving yourself the right amount will come naturally.

Follow the 20-minute rule. Think you're still hungry? Wait 20 minutes before going for a second serving. Studies show it takes about 20 minutes for the brain to get the message that you're full so wait it out a bit.

Learn the difference between REAL FOOD and FAKE FOOD.

Here are a couple of general rules on this.

- If nature didn't make it, it's not real food.
- If it's in a jar, packet, or box, it may be real food but it's been processed so much that you might as well forget it because there's hardly any nutrients left. (Plus, added salt and sugar!)
- If there's something on the nutritional label that you can't pronounce, don't buy it.

Don't buy food, cook food.

We leave in a world where everything is ready-made. It may be convenient but it also means we no longer have control over what we put in our mouths. However, do you really want food manufacturers to dictate what you eat? Take back your power by cooking your own food!

Also, buying cooked food or ready-to-eat meals come with a lot of salt, fat, and sugar. If you cook at home, you can avoid all of these. Here are some tips.

- **Steam vegetables.** When was the last time you were served 'virgin' side dishes in a restaurant? (The answer: never.) Steaming veggies at home means you get their full nutritional value, especially if you don't overcook them.
- **Don't deep-fry; bake, grill, or roast instead.** You already know deep-fried stuff is not good for you. Plus, if you bake, grill, or roast at home you have control over what marinade or sauce to use. (Go for low-fat liquids like broth, lemon juice, or even wine.)
- **Buy fish whole.** Not only is buying and steaming a whole fish more cost-effective, but it's also healthier because you skip all salt, sugar, and oil that come with pre-cooked or ready-to-eat fish meals.
- **Shop and cook with the changing seasons.** Buying foods in season is (1) healthier, (2) cheaper, (3) tastes better because they were not forced to ripen, and (4) it's pretty exciting to look forward to the different foods that each season brings!

How to Know If Your Body Is Getting Better

How do you know if the zero sugar diet is working for you? Although you can measure and keep track of your weight (after all, you just need a weight scale for that), I urge you to also take note of the many positive, healthy, life-altering changes that will happen while you're on this diet.

> **You DON'T automatically reach out for unhealthy foods anymore.**
> Although it may be very hard to believe now, your desire for most of your current 'go-to' food items will disappear. While on the zero sugar diet, you'll learn techniques that will BREAK certain sugar addiction habits. As a result, you won't just instinctively reach for that cookie.
>
> Weight loss alters your taste buds.[16] As you lose weight, your craving for certain food items will reduce or even disappear. Ever heard of formerly obese people gagging at the thought of eating foods they gorged on before? Well, that's all true and you'll experience it too.

> **You DON'T think of food as an automatic reward for something anymore.** From a very young age, we've been given food as a reward for something (e.g., good behavior, good grades, etc.). The minute you go for something else rather than food as a treat or prize for something great that happened to you - mark that event. That's one of the signs this diet is working for you.

> **You sleep better and wake up differently.**
> Is tossing and turning in bed now a thing of the past? That's because weight loss is linked to improved sleep quality[17]. It's also related to a reduction in the occurrence of sleep apnea, a serious sleep disorder wherein you stop breathing at various intervals during sleep.
>
> And guess what? Experiencing good quality sleep means you wake up refreshed, rejuvenated, and energized. This means no more dragging your feet out of bed, and struggling to find the energy to cope during the day.

> **Your hair and skin look different.**
> It's not hype when someone says that you seem to be 'glowing' now that you've kicked sugar out of your life. As mentioned before, you are what you eat.
>
> While you're on the zero sugar diet, the focus is on REAL FOOD that nourishes your entire body. And while not everyone will notice the positive changes inside your body, they won't be able to help but notice the differences outside it. The

changes are primarily because of the vitamins and minerals you're now consuming. Also – water!

Water helps maintain clear skin and improve its elasticity, contributing to your younger look. In fact, drinking just two (2) cups of water can increase blood flow to your skin, giving it an even tone.

Water also reduces that 'puffy' look. Contrary to popular belief, puffiness is not a sign of excess water. It's a sign of dehydration!

When you're dehydrated, your skin KEEPS water. When you do drink enough water, your skin will 'let go' of this excess water and so your face will lose that swelling. puffy, or bloated look.

> **You'll be more mobile.**
Additional weight puts a lot of pressure on the knees and joints. In a 2012 study of adults with obesity and Type 2 diabetes, researchers found that as little as a 1% drop in weight made the subjects more mobile by over 7%![18]

So don't be surprised if things you thought were impossible for you to do before suddenly seem conceivable now.

> **You may find yourself not needing your meds.**
As you lose weight, your overall health improves. As a result, you may be able to take lower doses of your current medications or stop taking them altogether. That's a lot of savings for you! (As always, please check with your physician before you make any changes to your medications.)

> **You'll be more at peace with everything around you.**
Bad food means a bad mood. So many nasty chemicals are triggered in your brain due to bad and unhealthy food choices. Also, the constant sugar highs and lows do nothing for your mood. Hyper one moment, hangry (hungry + angry) the next is never attractive, no?

Overweight people also have a lot of insecurities[19] that are often masked as anger at everything and everyone. A deep sense of failure and unworthiness is also pretty common.

However, as you banish sugar and lose weight you'll find yourself calmer, more relaxed, and more accepting of things and people around you.

➤ **Ok, your OLD clothes DON'T fit anymore!**

There is nothing to add to this, is there?

Chapter 4

Zero Sugar Diet Battle Plan

C HOOSING a healthy eating, healthy living lifestyle is one of the best decisions you'll ever make in your life. Many people do this but sadly, many people fail too because they are not armed with the right knowledge.

The following are practical, doable, REAL LIFE techniques to help you navigate certain crossroads you will definitely encounter in this journey.

7 Tips to Curb Your Sweet Tooth

Yes, resisting the urge to grab something sinfully sweet is hard but, repeat after me...IT CAN BE DONE!

1.   **Brush your teeth.** Yep, when the craving hits, get up... and brush your teeth. Floss even! By altering the taste in your mouth, you shift your perspective. Also, have you ever tried to consume something immediately after brushing? The food or drink does not taste nice, no? This will serve to 'turn you off' those cravings sooner than you think.

2.   **Water is your new best friend.** Are you hungry or thirsty? Believe it or not, it's sometimes hard to differentiate between a need for food and a need for hydration.

     This is because even a tiny amount of dehydration can activate the hypothalamus to turn on both the hunger and thirst centers of our brains. Drinking enough water is one of the easiest ways to keep sugar cravings at bay. Further, water consumption cuts down the chance of you reaching out for unhealthier beverages.

     10 Tips to Drink More Water!

     Believe it or not, many people find it hard to increase their water intake. You've probably already heard of the **8x8 rule** (eight 8-ounce glasses of water per day). That's just about two (2) liters of water. However, during a weight loss journey, it's recommended to increase this intake to three (3) liters per day, and a lot of people find this difficult.

     •   **Start your day with water.**
         When you wake up, start your day with a glass of lukewarm water (a slice of lemon in it wouldn't hurt either). Not only will this re-hydrate you after

HOURS of zzzzz's but it's also a great way to stave off bingeing on the wrong type of breakfast.

- **Get an engaging water bottle.**

  Ok, this is personal. I've seen some grown-up women carry water bottles with designs of their favorite cartoon characters when they were little... in PINK! I say, good for you! Whatever it takes, right?

  However, if you don't want to go the nostalgic way, how about just the practical way? For instance, get a water bottle that's 'marked' with the different hours of the day so that you're reminded that you should drink a certain amount of water by, say, noon. (You can also just get an old water bottle and use a marker and write these hours down yourself.)

- **Get some rubber bands and put this around your drinking bottle.**

  Each time you finish, remove a rubber band from your drinking glass or bottle. Fill up and keep ongoing throughout the day till you remove all the rubber bands.

- **Flavor your water.**

  I get it; water can be so boring! Liven things up by slicing different fruits and putting them in your water. Lemon, mint, and ginger are personal favorites of mine. But feel free to experiment!

- **Spice it up.**

  Try eating spicy food that's BEYOND your comfort zone. It's guaranteed to make you reach for a glass of water. And you don't need to go out for this either. Start adding chili flakes, cayenne pepper, etc. to your dishes to up the ante. (This is great for your metabolism too!)

- **'Eat' water.**

  Snack on watermelons, cucumbers, celery, and so on.

- **1:1**

  Dining out or having an evening out? Drink a glass of water for every alcoholic and/or non-alcoholic beverage you consume.

- **Make water your 24/7 companion.**

  Make your water glass or bottle as close a companion as your mobile phone! Hey, if you carry it around, might as well make actual use of it, right?

- **High-tech it.**

  Download a water tracker app; preferable one that's constantly - irritatingly (i.e., something that constantly beeps till you take a sip of water).

- **End your day with water.**

  After brushing your teeth, grab a glass of water and drink. Bring the empty glass to your nightstand because, you know... you need it for tomorrow morning's first water sip :)

3. **Don't grab food, grab something inspirational.** One of the best ways to fight sugar cravings is to flood your mind with health and fitness-related inspiration instead.

   For example, have you been taking notes of your weight loss journey? If you have, go and review your progress. See how far you've come. Be proud of that. Now is not the time to sabotage your progress, no?

   Another example is to immediately grab a fitness magazine or visit a health and fitness website. Basically, instead of focusing on the craving, you're negating that by re-focusing on your health.

4. **Learn the art of 'healthy substituting'.**

   When the craving kicks – give in. However, give in with healthy substitutes!

   10 Healthy Substitutes for Common Snack Cravings

   - **Chocolate -> Dark chocolate.**

     Switch to organic dark chocolate (at least 70% pure). Dark chocolate is rich in nutrients and contains fiber, iron, magnesium, copper, potassium, phosphorus, zinc, and selenium. It's also rich in antioxidants.

- **Chips -> Baked sweet potato wedges; multi-grain flatbread with hummus**
  Sweet potatoes are rich in beta-carotene and have been proven to raise levels of vitamin A in our blood. They're also full of vitamins A[20], B6, C, and D. Vitamin B6 has been linked to helping decrease the concurrence of heart attacks and certain degenerative diseases. (Click here for a Baked Sweet Potato Wedges recipe.)

- **Ice cream -> frozen, naturally-flavored flavored Greek yogurt.**
  Did you know that ice cream is basically churned frozen fat and sugar? Not good at all for healthy eating! Frozen yogurt, on the other hand, contains low levels of both and contains probiotics to help promote gut health. However, you will undo your good intentions if you flavor your yogurt with unhealthy food choices. The best is to mix it with fresh fruit and/or nuts. (Click here for a Greek yogurt ice cream recipe.)

- **Beer -> Red wine**
  Beer is high in calories. Depending on the type of beer, it can be anywhere from 200 to 400 per pint. The better alternative, if you must, is red wine, which has approximately 100-120 calories per glass. Red wine has also been linked to flavonoids, which may protect your skin from harmful UV rays.[21] Resveratrol in red wine may also reduce the effects of aging.

- **Hamburger -> Grilled chicken patty**
  The standard burger is about 350 calories. Grill a big, 150-gram piece of chicken breast, and you only consume 220 calories.

- **Pizza -> Whole wheat pita pockets.**
  Pizza, with its thick dough (starch!), layers of cheese (fat!), and unhealthy toppings (fat and salt!) may be delish but it's not healthy. Get the same satisfaction for less health damage with whole wheat pita bread stuffed with spicy grilled chicken, crunchy veggies, and a yogurt-based dressing.

- **Chips -> Popcorn**
  Potato chips, or any crisps for that matter, are loaded with salt and saturated fat. The problem too is that research has shown that consuming a very salty snack makes you crave and eat fatty foods in general, thus promoting weight gain.[22] So replace crisps with plain popcorn instead. They are full of antioxidants, fiber, and are low in calories.

  However, don't buy the flavored, buttered, already-popped variety as they contain a lot of salt and saturated fat too! Go for the unpopped corn kernels and pop them yourself.

- **Cake -> Whole wheat, organic banana bread**
  Cakes. Butter, flour, sugar... by now, you know this is not healthy eating, healthy living food. However, not all cakes are bad at all! Try this whole wheat, organic banana bread instead. It's rich in fiber and the whole wheat flour contains potassium, magnesium, and zinc.

- **Instant Noodles -> Homemade miso soup with buckwheat noodles**
  Apart from being salt city, a packet of instant noodles contains approximately 350 to 400 calories, plus about 14 grams of fat. Another problem is that instant noodles contain high levels of monosodium glutamate (MSG), a flavor enhancer that has been linked to having toxic effects on the body.[23]

  Try a homemade miso soup with buckwheat noodles instead. (Click here for a Miso Soup with Buckwheat Noodles recipe.) It's A LOT lower in calories. Plus, miso soup is known to have *A. oryzae*, a probiotic that's linked to lowering the risk of inflammatory bowel disease and other gut issues.

- Cookie -> No-Bake Chocolate Cookie

  Cookies. Butter, flour, sugar... They're just like cake - but harder. Reach for no-bake cookies instead. They are much lower in calories and since they're no-bake, they're easy to whip up too! (Click here for a No-Bake Chocolate Cookie recipe.)

5. **Break the pattern.**

Most of the time, a craving is triggered by something. So instead of reacting automatically, by grabbing whatever it is you're craving, pause and ANALYZE the situation.

- **What's the trigger?**

  Do you crave something every time you sit with your partner at the end of the day to unwind? If so, find an alternative non-food way to connect with your partner. This could simply be talking about each other's day, playing a board game or a hand of cards, or just talking about the kids and making plans.

  This is also a great opportunity to influence your partner to be healthier. For instance, instead of watching TV after dinner, encourage your partner to join you for a walk instead.

- **PAUSE and find out what you really need.**

  A craving is sometimes not a need for food, but something else. Perhaps you're just thirsty, or you're unconsciously trying to put off doing something. Reflect and act on what you really need – not on the craving.

6. **Reach out – to your support group.**

Don't reach out for food, reach out for support. When you're going through something, you don't need a lecture, you need emotional support. So when a bad craving hits, hit up family, friends, colleagues, or an online support group who have gone through the same journey before.

They will understand better because they've already been through what you're going through. They will also be more equipped to help you overcome your cravings by giving 'been there, done that' advice, tips, or simply just by being there for you.

A Note About Lack of Support from Family and Close Friends

It's not uncommon to not get the help, support, and understanding you need from your immediate circle. Please have it in your heart not to blame them.

Firstly, **they don't want to lose you**. Food is a symbolic, social activity. We eat with family and friends to bond together. So a shift in how you see food may be extremely hard for them to understand. Most of the time though, it's really not about not wanting you to be healthy. It's about not understanding why you don't want to bond with them anymore.

Sadly though, this inability to understand you creates a situation where your healthy eating, healthy living attempts get sabotaged. For instance, your partner KNOWS you're trying to avoid late-night snacking and here he goes bringing out a sugar buffet of snacks.

Secondly, **they lack 'healthy eating' knowledge**. As you've read in this guide, sugar addiction is not just about sugar per se. It's about habits. It's about routine. It's about not knowing what sugar is doing to your body. It's about mindset. It's about knowing what to do to kick sugar to the curb.

#1   Greek Yogurt Ice Cream So much knowledge is in your hands now; knowledge they don't have. As such, they don't understand, and thus can't support, the changes you want to make.

Thirdly, **they may be jealous of you**. Oftentimes, it's not just you struggling with weight and sugar addiction in your immediate circle. And any success you gain in your journey pricks at their conscience because now... you're leaving them behind.

So, the all-important question -> **what do you do?**
And here's the all-important answer -> **Live your life the way you want it!**

Remember that even though you understand why they may not or cannot support you, it doesn't mean that you should conform to what *they* want.
YOUR BODY. YOUR HEALTH. YOUR LIFE.
Don't follow them. Let them follow you!

7.   **Wait for it to pass.** Sugar cravings come and go. The key is to wait it out. So the next time you feel the need for a sugar rush, hit pause. Take a deep breath and let it out slowly. Stand up and do something else. Ignore it. Yes, you can!

12 Sugar Addiction Battle Strategies
It's great to know how NOT to give in when sugar cravings hit, but isn't it better to avoid cravings altogether? You bet it is!

Here are 12 techniques to adapt to put a STOP to roller coaster cravings and binges.

#1   **Eat MINDFULLY.**

What does it mean to eat mindfully? I get this question a lot. Is it about meditating before you put any morsel of food in your body? No.

Mindful eating is about AWARENESS. Great! But how does that prevent sugar cravings and food addiction?

When you sit down to eat a meal, don't just chug it down. Take your time. Avoid distractions such as watching TV while you eat or staring blindly at your mobile device. You need to be in the moment to appreciate food and be satiated by it. And science supports this.

One study with binge eaters showed mindful eating lowered binge eating incidents from 4 to 1.5 times per week![24]

So basically, if you're MINDFUL or AWARE of food and how it nourishes your body, it's not likely that you will just go and grab something unhealthy.

5 Tips to Practice Mindful Eating

a)   Eat and chew slowly.
b)   Don't rush meals. Eating is not a contest.
c)   Focus on the food or meal itself and ask yourself why it's a healthy choice.
d)   Focus on the company. (Preferably eat meals with others.)
e)   Before going for another serving, ask yourself first if you're REALLY still hungry.

#2   **Know your CRAVE O'CLOCK.**
We are creatures of habit. As you keep a food journal or simply take note of meal times and 'crave times', a pattern will emerge. If it's the dreaded 'post-lunch slump' of 'afternoon dip' – don't eat, take a nap! Studies show that taking afternoon naps boosts productivity[25] anyway so win-win!

#3   **Stock up on veggies.** Fibrous vegetables are low in calories and high in nutrients and fiber so they fill you up longer, without introducing added calories into your system. Fruits and whole grains are of course healthy too but they are also rich in calories and usually have a higher glycemic load than their green, leafy counterparts. The moral lesson? Get most of your carbs from vegetables, and you PREVENT sugar cravings.

#4   **Stop looking at 'food porn'.** We are constantly bombarded with food pictures online. So to prevent cravings from being triggered, avoid looking at food porn. If you must, then have a go-to list of websites and social media resources that focus on providing low carbohydrate, zero sugar food.

#5   **Hit the sack and get enough good-quality Zzzzzz.**
Sleep deprivation is linked to higher levels of body fat and appetite. Lack of good quality sleep also hinders cognitive function such as problem-solving, attentiveness, reasoning, and concentration. When you don't get enough sleep, you don't feel energized. You feel tired, grumpy, and hungry. And when you feel like this, your tendency is to crave foods high in sugar to artificially generate energy.

#6   **Learn techniques to overcome stress.** Life is full of stress - big and small. That's a given. Sadly, oftentimes, stress can lead to cravings. Somehow, somewhere, food has become a coping mechanism. So, let's learn some new ways to cope with the stress that has nothing to do with food.

15 Non-Food Related Ways to Deal with Every Stress

1.   **BREATHE**. Deep breathing is one of the easiest and fastest ways to get rid of stress. When you breathe deeply, a message is sent to your brain to calm down and relax. The brain then sends this 'calm down' message to your body.
2.   Read a **book**.
3.   Play restful, **calming music** (e.g., rain, sounds of nature, etc.)
4.   **Take a walk.**
5.   Do **yoga**.
6.   Take a 5- or 10-minute **meditation break**.
7.   Take a **bath**.
8.   Light a scented candle and **sit in silence**.
9.   Go to YouTube and **watch funny videos**. Home videos, baby videos, animal videos, anything that will make you laugh.
10.   Look at **family vacation pictures** or any picture that makes you feel happy. The point is to remind yourself of a happy point in your life to put your current stress into perspective.
11.   Get your journal and **start writing** down (instead of acting on) your feelings. Journaling is a very powerful way to get rid of stress.

    Many of the anti-stress tips here are about re-focusing the attention of your mind and body away from stress. Journaling, on the other hand, gives you a way to address stress directly.

For instance, you may want to shout at someone when stressed. Now, we both know that you might regret this action later so instead of ACTING on this urge, simply WRITE DOWN what you want to say to that person instead.

12.   **Dance!** If the environment permits, play your favorite dance tune as loud as you can and stomp and shake the stress away.

13.   **Call someone.**

14.   **Work out.** Exercise releases endorphins, the happy hormone, and as such naturally reduces stress![26]

15.   Don't ever forget this mantra – **THIS TOO WILL PASS.**

#7   **Eat more often.** It may sound counter-intuitive but spacing your meals every three or four hours prevents your blood sugar levels from dipping. As a result, you don't have those 'hunger pangs' and you won't reach out for a cookie for a 'quick fix'.

#8   **Spinach supplement, anyone?** Spinach supplements are now on the market and studies show that consuming 3.7–5 grams of spinach extract during meal times may lower appetite and cravings for several hours.[27]

#9   **Turn to vitamins.** If you're on a diet, chances are you may be lacking some important vitamin or mineral. This deficiency can also trigger the brain to activate its craving center so that you take in more food. The best way to handle this is to consult a physician before you start your weight loss journey, and come up with a nutrition supplementation program to ensure you consume everything that your body needs.

#10 **You've got to move it, move it.** It is often said that you don't need to exercise to lose weight.[28] However, it's such a GREAT way to boost insulin sensitivity and speed up your metabolism. It may not be needed to lose weight but it's definitely needed to be fit and to tone your body. And yes, it helps beat cravings!

#11 **Avoid boredom.** Oftentimes, sugar cravings are the result of boredom. Yes, there's such a thing as 'boredom eating'. There are two things you can do to avoid boredom.

Firstly, plan your days to a T. Grab your calendar, appointment notebook, or simply use your mobile phone and plan out every single hour of your day. This activity is called **block timing**. Keep in mind that you shouldn't fill your hours and days with just major events. The point is to plan and schedule everything so that there's absolutely no time to get bored.

For example, if you're usually free (and bored) after dinner till bedtime, then consider this.

> *Monday night: laundry!*
> *Tuesday night: new hobby (e.g., cross-stitch, bullet journaling, etc.)*
> *Wednesday night: call mom/brother/sister/friend/colleague*
> *Thursday night: read a book or learn a new exercise routine*
> *Friday night: me time (at least 1 hour soak in the tub; candles and all)*
> *Saturday night: meal prep*
> *Sunday night: plan coming week*

Secondly, adopt a nighttime walk routine. Many people who can't find the time to exercise during the day find that walking at night enables them to get some movement in, and perhaps more importantly, enables them to have some ME time and reflect.

#12 **Don't go to the supermarket hungry!** When you're hungry while you do your grocery shopping, chances are you'll make unhealthy food choices. We go back again to that *instant gratification* or *instant fulfillment* we think we get by consuming high-calorie, sugar-laden food. Instead, have a 'shopping game plan' and stick to it.

Firstly, always have a grocery shopping list with you. Make it a habit to make your grocery list on a certain day (e.g., Sunday) and make it a habit to shop a certain day as well (e.g., Tuesday). This habit forces you to keep stock of what you have in-house and list only what you need for the week. When you shop, bring the list, and stick to it!

Secondly, know the layout of your grocery store. Once you know this, avoid all the 'unhealthy aisles', which are usually the middle aisles. When you enter the grocery store, spend most of your time on the produce section. This way, even if you're tempted to go to the middle aisles – you don't have time for it.

By the way, there's also research that hunger promotes the purchase of even non-food items.[29] So unless you need yet another potholder, don't shop hungry!

A Note on Dining Out and Handling Special Events

Going on a zero sugar diet doesn't mean you should skip going out altogether or miss important life events. As with grocery shopping, all you need is a game plan to address such situations.

- **Find out where you're eating out in advance.** Check out the menu beforehand, seek out the healthier options, and order these instead. Also, avoid consuming complementary food items set on the table such as breadsticks, salted nuts, white bread, and others as these are usually high-calorie, high-sugar food items. Opt to drink water with your meals too.

- **Go for appetizers.** Instead of ordering an appetizer and a main, consider ordering two appetizers instead. Also, ask for dressings on the side.

- **Ask for a healthy swap.** Luckily, many restaurants cater to healthy options nowadays, so instead of potato mash, ask if you can have a 'virgin' (nothing on it) baked sweet potato instead. Instead of white rice, ask for brown rice. If anything comes with a sauce, ask it to be served on the side.

- **Party time?** If you're going to a party where you KNOW there will be almost nothing but pizza, beer, and chips, then do the following: (1) Eat a light meal at home. (2) Arrive fashionably late! (3) DO NOT stand around the food table. (4) Socialize through conversion, not eating.

- Practice mindful eating.

- **Skip dessert.** Order black coffee or herb-infused tea and have a small piece of dark chocolate instead.

Clean Out Your Pantry, Freezer, and Refrigerator

Out of sight, out of mind. One of the best ways to succeed with your zero sugar diet is to simply remove temptation in your own house. After all, you can't deny yourself something, that's not there, right?

In one study, it was learned that people who had high-calorie foods within arm's reach are likely to weigh more than people who kept a bowl of fruit in their kitchens. [30] So to prevent any 'lapses', it's best if you clear out your pantry, freezer, and refrigerator of unhealthy food items before you embark on your zero sugar diet.

Look, chances are these places are up for some cleaning anyway; so take this as the perfect opportunity to declutter and organize these spaces.

As you go through these areas, you may find it hard to get rid of certain food items. You may even find it wasteful. However, remember this - your weight loss and health goals are far more important than holding onto comfort foods.

Think of it this way, you're not being wasteful. You're just getting rid of items that are making you sick.

Also, the goal is not just to empty your pantry, freezer, and refrigerator but to replenish them with items that you will need on hand during your zero sugar diet. As you will learn in Chapter 7, a zero sugar diet calls for making your own meals. Don't worry! All the recipes are easy and for beginners. You don't need to be a master chef to make them.

However, you'll soon realize that a new world of ingredients may be in order. And since you're just starting out, you may find it annoying to not have something in stock just when you're in the mood to meal prep. So, cleaning out your kitchen NOW is the perfect time to do it.

Tackling your refrigerator. Take everything out and give your refrigerator a good scrubbing (water + vinegar + washcloth will do).

What NOT to bring back: salad dressings, jams, soft drinks, and anything else that's high in calories and loaded with sugar.

Instead fill your ref with zero sugar essentials like cottage cheese, Greek yogurt, fruits, and vegetables. No time to dice and chop? Make life easier and buy pre-cut veggies and fruit.

Tackling your pantry. Same as with your refrigerator, take everything down and give your cupboards a good wipe. White bread, white rice, pasta, boxed macaroni and cheese, boxed breakfast cereals, bottled sauces... they all need to go. Don't be surprised if you find out there's hardly anything to put back.

In fact, I want you to take a big step back and STARE at all the items you're going to let go of. These are the things making you sick, fat, unhealthy, and unhappy. Be glad to let them go! And be excited about what you're going to replace them with.

Tip: For added 'excitement', think of recycling old jars or get some inexpensive transparent containers. Seeing your new food items on display can give such a healthy kick and can be a real inspiration to get creative in the kitchen.

Tackling your freezer. Take out all freezer-burned items, frozen cakes and pastries, frozen dinners, frozen pizza, frozen snacks (I see you frozen cheese pockets!), and ice cream. What to bring back: frozen chicken, beef, fish, pork, and any other unprocessed meat option.

Although fresh is best, frozen fruits and vegetables are also great options to have in there. Frozen veggies can be quickly made into a great and healthy side dish, and frozen fruit can be quickly added to any healthy, energy-boosting smoothie.

Still not sure about what to clear out and what to keep? Here's a low-sugar kitchen list to guide you.

HOW TO STOCK A LOW-SUGAR KITCHEN	
Clear Out	**Swap With**
Artificial sweeteners	Sugar/Stevia
Breakfast cereal	Oatmeal
Candy, dried fruit snack	Dark chocolate
Canned beans	Dried beans
Canned fruit	Fresh or frozen fruit
Canned vegetables	Fresh or frozen vegetables
Chip and crackers	Raw nuts (unsalted)
Crisps, chips	Popcorn
Egg substitutes	Eggs!
Fat-free yogurt	Greek yogurt
Flavored yogurt	Greek yogurt
Frozen dinners	Fresh meals
Fruit juice	Fruit-infused water
Margarine	Butter (preferably grass-fed)

Non-fat or skim milk	Whole milk
Processed cheese	Natural cheese (e.g., mozzarella, feta, cottage cheese)
Processed, canned meat	Lean cuts of meat
Protein or fiber bars	Fresh meals
Ready-made salad dressing	Homemade olive oil and lemon dressing
Soft drinks and sports drinks	Water, seltzer
Vegetable oil/canola oil	Olive oil / Avocado oil / Extra-virgin olive oil
White bread	Sprouted bread
White pasta	Chickpea pasta
White rice	Brown rice

Tip: For the first few days of your zero sugar diet, it's best to have zero temptations in-house. Later on, you can buy tempting foods or snacks but then keep them on a higher shelf or anywhere that's NOT within easy reach.

Think Beyond Your Kitchen

Don't just focus on what's inside your kitchen. There are other ways you can support your new healthy eating, healthy living lifestyle.

Herb garden, anyone? Instead of buying dried herbs, why not have a steady supply of them by getting the real stuff? This saves money and you end up with a new hobby!

Go to your local garden nursery and select a few basic herbs to start with such as mint (natural breath freshener), basil (must-have in any pasta sauce), rosemary, thyme, and oregano. Go back home and re-pot or replant them in your garden. But if you're not up for a full garden just yet then just keep the pots on your windowsill or anywhere they can get ample sunshine. Take care of them and you'll be fully rewarded in turn!

Revisit your cookbooks. Dust off the cookbook shelf and get rid of (or store) anything related to baking and sugar. Instead, focus on cookbooks about healthy recipes. If you don't have any, no problem. No need to buy either. Just go online and start bookmarking healthy recipes and make a deal with yourself to try at least one new zero-sugar recipe each week.

Improve your spice rack. On average, spices last up to three to four years. Anything longer should be thrown out. The exciting part now is replenishing your spice rack not just with new ones but with spices you've never tried before. After all, variety is the *spice* of life.

Weight Loss and Weight Maintenance

Losing weight is only half the battle. Maintaining your weight loss is the other half. The secret is to permanently adopt the healthy eating, healthy living activities you used during the diet.

A very low carbohydrate, zero sugar diet is used to jumpstart weight loss and break sugar's addictive claim on your mind and body. Once you've achieved this, you can slowly re-integrate carbs and sugar back into your diet.

However, it's imperative that you only add back COMPLEX CARBS and NATURAL SUGARS. Otherwise, you'll just be undoing all your hard work!

Check your calories. As mentioned before, with a zero sugar diet, you *automatically* decrease your calorie intake. However, for weight loss maintenance, it's a good idea to know how many calories you need to maintain your achieved weight.

There are many factors that affect your required calorie intake such as your age, gender, ethnicity, activity levels, and so on. You can use an online calculator to arrive at your daily caloric requirements. However, it's best to consult your physician.

Keep up the protein intake. Protein has been associated with improved metabolism, lower appetite, and supports certain weight-regulating hormones.[31] By continuing to focus on protein in your diet, you lower *ghrelin* (the hunger hormone) and improve *leptin* (the satiety hormone) in your body.

Also, protein takes more to break down in the body than carbs or fat. It's said that protein has a thermic effect of 20-30%, compared to carbs at 5-10%, and fat at 0-3%.[32] Protein is also believed to be great at suppressing cravings.

The bottom line is this: keep on focusing that you consume enough protein during meals for weight loss maintenance.

Weigh yourself regularly. This is a personal thing. Some people swear by it, while others claim to be stressed out by it. I say use it. Why? It's better to notice micro-changes in your weight so you don't overreact and overcompensate by making unhealthy and unsafe decisions such as skipping a meal.

Try to weigh yourself at the same time and day each week. However, choose 'weighing day' wisely. For instance, if Sunday is a family day celebrated with a BIG lunch or dinner, then skip Monday as your 'weighing day'. After such a meal, you're

bound to be a bit heavier the following day. That's OK. You can't have the EXACT same weight every single day. Slight fluctuations occur. That's fine.

So, choose your day and make it a habit to weigh yourself AFTER your morning bathroom rituals (but before your first meal of the day). If the scale says you're a bit heavier then take action by being more mindful of your food choice for a day or two.

The bottom line is this: treat the weighing scale as a useful tool, not an enemy.

Don't go back to the dark side. You've worked so hard. Wow, you! To *maintain* your weight, keep true to the healthy eating, healthy living principles you applied to *lose* weight.

MOVE ON. This is perhaps one of the best tips I can give you on weight loss maintenance. Many dieters fall prey to the thinking of 'going back' to old ways now that they've achieved their desired weight. On the contrary, what you should do is leave all that behind.

And it's not just about using the same techniques you learned to lose weight. It's about discovering NEW ways to motivate you on this road of healthy living.

Here are some examples:
- You learned that a support group can have a big, positive impact on your weight loss -> move on to supporting someone else.
- You learned how to set up a low-sugar kitchen -> move on to attending a low-sugar cooking class.
- You learned about smart food swaps -> move on to take complete stock of your life and see what other, better swaps you can do.

Chapter 5
A New Way of Eating = A New Way of Living

Identify Your 'DAY 1'

You got the Healthy Eating for Healthy Living guide. That's a life-changing decision. Now it's time to further act on that decision by concretely deciding EXACTLY WHEN you should start your zero sugar life.

Some people just know that NOW is the perfect time. If you're one of them, go right ahead and complete this sentence.

I AM GOING TO START MY ZERO-SUGAR DIET ON: _____

Writing down an exact date is good because **you're committing to this change**, not to anyone, but **to YOURSELF**.

However, if you're not sure when the perfect time is, perhaps the following tips can help you.

➢ **BEST 'DAY 1' TIP: After your birthday**
According to research from the University of Pennsylvania[33], the day after your birthday is a great day to start to make BIG changes such as embarking on a health journey. This is called the 'fresh start' effect that many people feel after going through a personal milestone.

➢ **BEST 'DAY 1' TIP: Monday**
Mondays symbolize the start of the week, and as such may also symbolize the start of a new you. Also, Mondays are practical for many people because weekends are usually when family gatherings, birthday celebrations, and friend get-togethers happen.

➢ **BEST 'DAY 1' TIP: Any day in October**
This may sound counter-intuitive. After all, the holidays are just around the corner so are you setting yourself for failure? According to research[34], not at all.

The holidays do tend to make people gain weight. However, by starting a weight loss or health journey in October, you give yourself the opportunity to lose weight *before* the holidays. So even if you do gain some weight, you end up weighing the same (pre-October) once January rolls in.

On another note, many people who start a zero sugar diet in October find that they don't overindulge during the holidays. Why?

Firstly, they love what they've accomplished health- and weight-wise so they find it easy to 'stay true' to their new eating lifestyles.

Secondly, just as you've learned in this eBook, they now have the skills to eat mindfully and choose healthy food so quite frankly, unhealthy holiday food temptations are just not as strong as they used to!

Meal Planning and Meal Prepping

Meal planning is when you think about, plan, and list down the snacks and meals you want to consume in advance, preferable over the coming week (7 days).

Now, depending on your schedule and personal preference, you can simply plan out your meals and prep and cook them the day you plan to eat them or prepare and cook everything in advance (e.g., over the weekend), freeze them, and then thaw and reheat over the week.

Regardless of what option you choose, **meal planning is key to a zero sugar diet**. This way, you remove any possibility of grabbing snacks or meals that don't fit your zero sugar, low carbohydrate lifestyle.

How to Meal Plan

Deciding what to eat every single day can be stressful. And oftentimes, because life gets in the way, healthy meals are sacrificed in favor of 'something easy'.

Meal planning takes away a lot of the stress and pressure associated with answering this simple question - what do we eat today?

So, here's how to meal plan.

1. Pick a day of the week that's less hectic for you (e.g., Saturday afternoon or evening).
2. Take out a notebook and write down the coming days of the week; Monday thru Sunday. (You can also use a kitchen whiteboard so everyone can see the week's menu.)
3. Break down each day to Breakfast, Morning Snack, Lunch, Afternoon Snack, Dinner, and Dessert.

4. Keeping your zero sugar, low carbohydrate goals in mind, write down everything you should be eating for EACH meal.

5. Create a grocery list for the week based on your meal plan and stick to that list. No extras for now.

The advantage of meal planning is that you give yourself enough time to determine what you want to eat for the coming week. No stress.

Also, meal planning helps you come up with the RIGHT variety of healthy meals. During a busy week, you may not be realizing that you're eating the same meals (e.g., chicken and rice) over and over.

However, if you meal plan, you can mindfully choose what to eat over the mix and come up with a good, healthy, and nutritious variation of chicken, fish, meat, and vegetable meals.

Here's another tip: go online and look for zero sugar recipes you've never tried before. Go to Pinterest and search for yummy low carbohydrate ideas. Find zero sugar online forums and see what people are finding delicious. Let yourself be inspired!

How to Meal Prep

Let's face it. Even with the best intentions, a stressful day, feeling tired or unplanned events can lead to opting for the fast and easy solution – takeout or drive-thru.

However, if you ALREADY have a tasty and healthy meal ready to be consumed... well, that's already 'fast food' right there!

Meal prepping is the next step to meal planning. It's acting on your healthy meal plans and intentions.

Meal prepping is when you prepare, cook, and portion out your emails in advance. Many people opt to make their meals on the weekend – Saturday or Sunday – and then put them in the freezer.

As the week progresses, you simply take out a frozen meal and let it thaw during the day or pop it directly in the microwave.

Is meal prepping tedious? It doesn't have to be!

Meal prepping can be a **fun family-bonding activity**. Get your partner and/or kids involved, and you just might be surprised at how much they like being a part of it.

Some people also like having **meal prepping get-togethers**, where a few friends cook together in large quantities and divide the resulting cooked food.

Whether you're doing it alone or with family and friends, here are some meal prepping methods for you:

- **Have ingredients ready-to-cook:** Cut, slice, and dice whatever you need for your planned meals. If necessary, steam, boil or bake them as well. On the day you need them, simply take them out of the fridge or freezer and cook away!

Example Recipe: Pasta Alla Norma

Ingredients:

2 eggplants, medium

1 onion, large

1 tbsp extra-virgin olive oil

2 cloves garlic, minced

1 can plum tomatoes

Salt and pepper to taste

Handful fresh basil (optional)

250 grams whole wheat or chickpea pasta

Directions:

1. **Weekend prep:** Pre-heat the oven to 200°C.
2. Chop the eggplants into bite-size pieces. Season it with salt and pepper and place them on a baking tray. (You can add other spices too such as oregano, chili flakes, etc.)
3. Bake the eggplants for 20-25 mins, tossing once.
4. In the meantime, chop the garlic and onion and put them into individual small containers.*
5. Take out the baked eggplants when done, cool, and refrigerate.
6. **Tuesday (or any weekday):** Cook the pasta as per package directions.
7. While waiting, sauté the pre-chopped garlic and onion until translucent.
8. Add the plum tomatoes. Season with salt and pepper.
9. Add the pre-baked eggplants and simmer until the pasta is cooked.
10. Add the pasta into the eggplant sauce. Toss and serve!

* Tip: If you use garlic and onion a lot in your meals, prepare a lot during the weekend and keep them (separately) in air-tight glass jars in the refrigerator. Saves a lot of time and stress during the week!

- **Make-ahead meals:** Prep and cook full meals over the weekend. Portion them out and freeze or refrigerate.

You can do this for the **Pasta Alla Norma** recipe above. Instead of cooking the whole meal on the day, you want to eat it. Cook the full meal on the weekend and simply reheat on the weekday.

- **Batch cooking:** This meal prepping method is great for meals that take longer to cook and use ingredients that freeze well.

For example, soups or meals that use beef take a long time to cook so instead of making just ONE family-sized portion, cook two or even three portions over the weekend. The meal can then be stored in the freezer and consumed over the coming weeks or even months.

- **Grab-and-go portions:** This method is great for snacks. Cut up A LOT of your favorite vegetables such as cucumbers, carrots, bell peppers, celery sticks, radishes, etc. Use a lunchbox or container with compartments and portion out a single serving of veggies, unsalted and unroasted nuts, and some fruit. Make a few of these grab-and-go treats to cover you over the weekdays. Handy AND healthy!

Figure out which meal prepping method suits you and your lifestyle and apply that one first. As you get more adept at meal prepping, trying the other methods should be easy.

As you may have noted above, meal prepping involves a lot of **FOOD STORING**.

Here are some tips on selecting the right storage containers.

- **Containers with compartments:** It's great if you can prep and put ingredients that belong to a specific meal together in one container. This means less searching for what you need when it's cooking time.

- **Airtight containers:** As you store ingredients and meals in the refrigerator, you don't want the various smells to co-mingle in there so it's best to keep them in airtight storage containers. Another advantage here is that they keep ingredients fresh and crisp longer.

- **Freezer-safe containers:** Prevent leakage, freezer burn, and loss of nutrients in your cooked meals by purchasing good-quality freezer-safe containers. Choose ones that stack well too to save freezer space.

- **BPA-free microwavable containers:** There's a lot of thawing and reheating when you meal prep so for your own health, invest in some quality BPA-free containers.

Lastly, to preserve the quality of planned meals and to prevent issues such as food poisoning, it's important to keep and reheat meals properly. Following are some important food safety standards from the USDA Food and Safety Inspection Service.[35]

✔ **Keep correct ref and freezer temperatures.**
Refrigerator temperatures should be kept at 5°C or below, while the freezer should be at -18°C) or below.

Tip: To be sure of refrigerator temps, get a fridge thermometer. They are inexpensive and help a lot in knowing the exact temperature of your refrigerator as you open and close it throughout the day.

Place the thermometer in different areas of your fridge every now and then to detect cold and warm spots. This way, you can position your food and drinks accordingly.

✔ **Cool foods before storing.**
After cooking certain ingredients or full meals, ensure you cool them down thoroughly before storing them. Cool them down fast by spreading them out on shallow containers and then pack and store them within two hours of cooking.

✔ **Label your meals,**
Apply a first in, first out approach to refrigerated cooked meals. This way, no meal is forgotten or stays longer in storage than it should. For this, it's best to label or mark your meals, i.e., write down the date you cooked the food.

✔ **Cook food to the right temperature.**
Invest in a food thermometer to ensure that food is cooked well. Most meats are cooked when their internal temperatures reach at least 75°C.

✔ **Thaw foods properly.**
When thawing prepared meals, it's best to take them out of the freezer a day ahead (or in the morning) and place them in the refrigerator. This enables the food to defrost slowly and safely (less chance for bacteria to be introduced). Further, slow thawing helps preserve food structure.

If time does not permit this, dip frozen foods completely in a big container with cold tap water. Replace the water every 30 minutes.

✔ **Reheat meals at the right temperature.**
Cooked meals should be reheated to 75°C. Frozen meals should be thoroughly thawed, reheated, and then consumed within 24 hours after being defrosted. Do not refreeze!

Here's another tip: **discover new ways to cook food.**

It seems that today's diet is all about deep-drying. But did you know that the way you cook your food has a direct impact on how food affects your health? Deep frying, in particular, can cause potentially toxic compounds to be released, which can lead to heart disease, cancer, and other illnesses.

Now that you're exploring meal planning and meal prepping, it's the perfect time to discover the joys of other cooking methods.

- **Baking** is when you prepare food using dry heat, without direct exposure to flames, typically using an oven.

  ### Healthy example: Baked Sweet Potato
  - Preheat oven to 200°C.
  - Wash a sweet potato to get rid of any dirt.
  - Using a fork, poke holes around the sweet potato.
  - Wrap it in aluminum foil and place it in the preheated oven.
  - Bake for 45-55 minutes.

  ### Healthy example: Chicken en Papillote
  - Preheat oven to 200°C.
  - Take two boneless, skinless chicken thighs and place them on parchment paper.
  - Add any vegetables you have in your fridge such as cherry tomatoes, zucchini, mushrooms, etc.
  - Drizzle with extra-virgin olive oil, and season with salt and pepper.
  - Bring the edges of the parchment paper to the center and fold them together tightly. Place the food packets on a sheet pan, and then place the sheet pan in the preheated oven.
  - Bake for 20-25 minutes.

- **Broiling** is when you prepare food using direct, high heat. It's different from baking or roasting in that the food is turned during the process (usually mid-way) to cook either side at a time.

- **Poaching** is when you prepare food by simmering it with a small amount of liquid.

  ### Healthy example: Poached Egg
  - Crack an egg into a small bowl. Set aside.
  - Bring a big pot of water to a boil, and then lower the heat to low.

- Add 1-2 tablespoons of vinegar to the water. Stir to create a vortex.
- Slowly add the egg to the middle of the vortex and cook it for 2-3 minutes.
- Using a slotted spoon, remove the egg and place it in some kitchen paper to remove any excess water.

- **Steaming** is when you prepare food by heating it in steam from boiling water. This is a great way of cooking vegetables as it preserves the flavor and a lot of its nutrients.

Healthy example: Steamed Green Beans

- Rinse the green beans and trim the edges.
- Put 1-2 inches of water in a medium to a large saucepan.
- Put a steamer basket on top of the saucepan, and place the green beans in the steamer basket.
- Bring the water to a boil. Reduce to medium-low, cover the saucepan, and steam the green beans for about 5 minutes.

*(Did you notice that we just made a whole meal with the **Chicken en Papillote**, **Baked Sweet Potato**, and the **Steamed Green Beans** recipes? Try it for dinner sometime!)*

- **Pressure cooking** is when you prepare food using a pressure cooker. This cooking method heats the air within a covered pot (the pressure cooker) to a very high temperature (above boiling point). This enables air pressure and steam to build up inside the cooking vessel, cooking food faster. As the pressure increases inside the pot, hot steam is compelled through the food to cook it thoroughly.

- **Simmering**, also known as the *moist heat method*, involves bringing water (or any liquid) to 85°C to 95°C (gentle bubbling) to cook food.

- **Stewing or slow cooking** is when you prepare food by subjecting it to a low temperature for a long period of time. Also known as the 'set it and forget it' cooking method, this technique is great for tendering tough meat cuts or when you simply don't have a lot of time to fuss in the kitchen. You can use either a slow cooker or your oven for this method.

- **Sous-vide** is when you prepare food by vacuum-sealing ingredients and immersing it in warm water. Just like slow cooking, it's a 'set it and forget it' cooking method. This is great for meal planning and prepping because you can pretty much put a whole meal in a vacuum pack, freeze it, and sous vide it during the week (without defrosting).

How to Shop for Healthy Food

Meal prepping starts with having healthy ingredients readily on hand in the kitchen. It's not surprising that changing your eating lifestyle also calls for a change in your grocery shopping habits. No worries though. I've got you covered with the following tips.

12 Tips to Help You Become Supermarket Savvy

1. Meal plan so that you can create an 'exact' grocery list.

    Tip: Don't just be a healthy shopper, be a savings savvy shopper too. Most grocery stores offer weekly discounts on certain food items. Focus on fresh produce, and keep this in mind when meal planning and creating your grocery list.

2. **Snack before you grocery shop.** When you're full, unhealthy food choices won't easily tempt you.

3. **Avoid free samples.** The supermarket is a breeding ground for many food marketers who want to introduce you to *What's New* in their assortment. Sadly, most of these concern highly manufactured food. So, skip the freebies and stay true to your low carbohydrate, zero sugar list.

4. **Send someone else to do the grocery shopping for you, preferably a man!** This may sound like an odd tip, but I swear it works. Men, in general, are not easily distracted by discounts, freebies, and free samples. They want to grab what's on the list and get out of there fast. So, if you know someone willing to do this for you – grab the opportunity.

5.   **Go for the rainbow.** Spend most of your time in the produce section and select fruits and vegetables of various colors. This is not just for aesthetics. The different colors represent the different vitamins and minerals you can get from each vegetable or fruit.

6.   **Avoid anything that comes in a box or package.** These food items normally mean 'processed'. So stay clear of these.

7.   **There's no shame in pre-cut fruits and veggies.** If time is an issue when it comes to meal planning and prepping, do yourself a favor and go for pre-cut produce. They may cost a bit more but if it saves you time and stress, why not?

8.   **Canned food can be good.** Fresh is best but canned food items such as tuna chunks in water and canned plum tomatoes are not bad at all. Just be sure you select canned food that's not processed with a ton of salt and sugar.

9.   **Avoid foods with hard-to-pronounce ingredients.** Real food is made up of easy-to-read and easy-to-understand ingredients. Once you see something on the label that's difficult to read or articulate, skip it.

10.   **Go beyond your local supermarket.** Instead of going to the supermarket, why not try and get the most of your week's supplies at the local farmer's market or food co-op? These places often offer the freshest seasonal produce, plenty of organic options, and many items sourced locally.

11.   **Buy in bulk.** If possible, stock up on healthy food choices so that you don't end up going to the supermarket often. For instance, whole grains like brown rice, steel-cut oats, dried beans, herbs and spices, and healthy snacks like popcorn can be bought in volume. This way, you don't need to constantly run to the supermarket and be tempted to grab something 'extra' on the way out.

   However, don't panic buy. If you buy anything in bulk, do so for items that you KNOW you would normally consume during your zero sugar diet.

12.   **Switch to using sustainable bags, crates, and/or containers.** Apart from being planet-friendly, having a *specific* set of grocery bags and containers helps you curb any unwanted buying. If something unhealthy won't fit in your bag anymore, it doesn't belong there.

Chapter 6
Gut Health - The Anti-Candida Cleanse

Various types of fungi live inside and outside the body. This includes the genus of yeasts called *Candida*. In small amounts, *candida* is not a problem at all. However, when this yeast propagates uncontrollably, it can result in a yeast infection called *candidiasis*.

Thrush (Oropharyngeal Candidiasis)

Candida overgrowth in the mouth and throat is called *thrush*. It's common in newborn babies, seniors, and people with weakened immune systems.

Vaginal Candidiasis

Candida overgrowth in the vagina is called *vaginal candidiasis* and an estimated 1.4 million outpatient visits for vaginal candidiasis happen yearly in the US.[36] At best, vaginal thrush is an itchy, irritating inconvenience. However, if not properly addressed, it can become recurrent and lead to severe inflammation, or a serious skin infection.

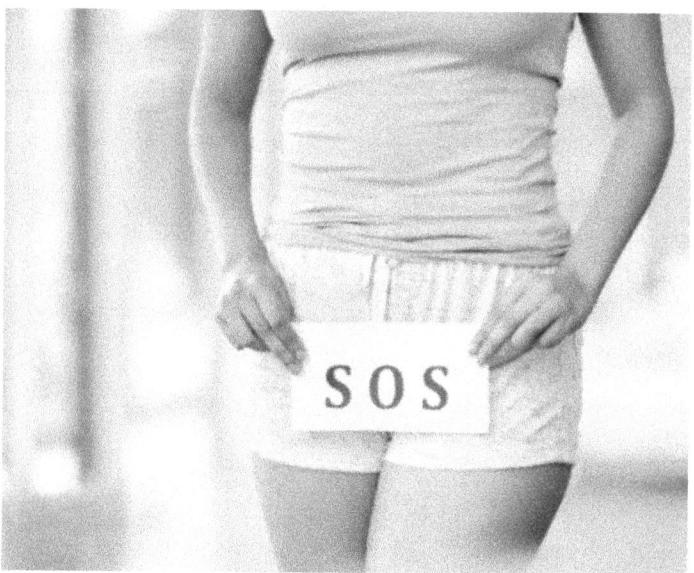

Invasive Candidiasis

No matter where the yeast infection starts, if not treated properly, candida yeast can enter the bloodstream. It can traverse the heart, brain, blood, eyes, and bones. It is this scenario – *invasive candidiasis* – that can lead to a dangerous, life-threatening infection.

With the many problems that Candida overgrowth presents, it's not surprising for a Candida cleanse to be in order now and them. In addition to gut health benefits, a Candida cleanse is also beneficial for the following:

- ✔   Better food digestion.
- ✔   Lower inflammation in the body.
- ✔   Improved mood.
- ✔   Higher energy levels.

So it's important to always keep *candida* growth at normal levels. To do this, you should be mindful of what triggers candida overgrowth.

One of the reasons *candida* can grow uncontrollably is too much consumption of sugar, refined carbs, and processed foods.[37]

Anti-Candida Cleanse

Candida is a yeast infection. Sugar is the primary fuel source of yeast. For this reason, an anti-candida cleanse focuses on limiting the intake of food items that promote yeast growth.

On such a cleanse, flour-based food items, grains, and sweeteners should be avoided. Fruit and starchy vegetable intake should also be limited to two servings daily.

Here are some of the food items to CONSUME on an anti-candida cleanse.

- ✔   Avocado
- ✔   Bone broth
- ✔   Coconut oil
- ✔   Cruciferous vegetables (broccoli, cauliflower, cabbage, Brussels sprouts)
- ✔   Dark chocolate
- ✔   Eggs
- ✔   Ginger
- ✔   Grass-fed beef
- ✔   Herbs
- ✔   Leafy greens

- ✔ Lemon
- ✔ Non-starchy vegetables
- ✔ Nuts
- ✔ Olive oil and olives
- ✔ Pasture-raised poultry, including chicken
- ✔ Rooibos, green tea
- ✔ Seeds (e.g., chia seeds, flaxseed, etc._
- ✔ Some kinds of fruit, including tomatoes and berries like strawberries and raspberries
- ✔ Spices
- ✔ Water
- ✔ Wild fish

Here are some of the food items to AVOID on an anti-candida cleanse.

- ✗ Alcohol, particularly beer and other beverages fermented or made with yeast
- ✗ Dairy
- ✗ Fermented foods (yogurt, kefir, kimchi, kombucha, and sauerkraut)
- ✗ Flour-based foods (e.g., donuts, cakes, bread, bagels, pizza, etc.)
- ✗ Mushrooms
- ✗ High-sugar foods
- ✗ High-sugar beverages
- ✗ Vinegar, including apple cider vinegar

A Note on Gluten

Gluten has been linked to gut problems, inflammation issues, and Candida overgrowth. For this reason, it's important to steer clear of white bread, white pasta, and most cereals containing gluten. Instead focus on gluten-free grains such as buckwheat, quinoa, and millet.

Luckily, non-starchy veggies are naturally gluten-free so you can simply substitute certain vegetables for grains. For example, cauliflower and broccoli can be used to make *cauliflower rice* and *broccoli rice*. (Note: if you don't want to make a 100% switch, then do 50% brown rice + 50% cauliflower rice.) You can also use zucchini as a pasta substitute. (Click here for a Cauliflower Rice recipe.)

Further, you can substitute most flours for gluten-free alternatives, such as almond flour, chickpea flour, buckwheat flour, or even oatmeal flour!

Chapter 7

The 7-Day Zero Sugar Diet Eating Plan

Recipes make or break a diet. If it's too restrictive or if the food items are way too different from what you would normally consume, chances are, you lower your chances of sticking to your diet.

If your diet is composed mainly of 'bland food' that you need to eat over and over again, you won't stick to your diet either!

This is why I made sure to offer you a variety of recipes that fit the following criteria: delicious, easy to prepare, and made from easy-to-find ingredients.

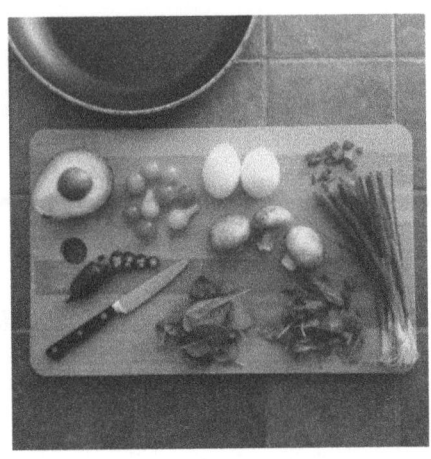

By easy-to-find, I mean that they are readily available at most local supermarkets. However, I do concede that you may not be familiar with some of these ingredients. And for those particular items, this is what I ask of you – **please keep an open mind.**

Just because you're not familiar with something, it doesn't mean you shouldn't try it. Take this as the perfect opportunity to GROW your mind and food experience

The recipes are broken down into Breakfast, Lunch, Dinner, and Dessert and Snacks. And each category has seven (7) recipes. This way, you'll have a different – something to look forward to – delicious meal for each day of the week!

IMPORTANT: If you have any allergies, please search online for substitutes.

Breakfast Recipes

Mom's right. Breakfast is the most important meal of the day. This is the time you fuel your body and give it the nourishment and energy it needs to tackle the day ahead strongly and confidently.

#1   Power Cereal

Ingredients:

1/2 cup almonds, chopped

1/2 cup walnuts, chopped

1/2 cup unsweetened coconut flakes

1 tbsp sesame seeds

1 tbsp. chia seeds

1/2 tsp. ground clove

1/2 tsp. ground cinnamon

1 tsp. pure vanilla extract

1/2 tsp. kosher salt

1 large egg white

1/4 cup coconut oil, melted

Directions:

1.   Preheat your oven to 180°C degrees.

2.   In a bowl, mix the almonds, walnuts, coconut flakes, sesame seeds, and chia seeds.

3.   Add the cloves, cinnamon, vanilla, and salt.

4.   In a separate bowl, beat the egg white until foamy. Stir this into the granola mixture.

5.   Add the melted coconut oil to the mixture.

6.   Lightly grease a baking sheet, and pour the mixture over it, spreading it into an even layer.

7.   Bake for 20- 25 mins, or until golden brown. Stir halfway through.

8.   Cool before serving.

#2   Veggie Hash Browns

Ingredients:

1 large egg

1/4 tsp. garlic powder

1 cup shredded cabbage

1/4 small yellow onion, thinly sliced

1 tbsp. extra-virgin olive oil (or coconut oil or avocado oil)

Salt and pepper to taste

Directions:

1.   Whisk together the egg garlic powder, salt, and pepper.

2.   Add the shredded cabbage and onion into the egg mixture. Stir just to combine.

3.   Heat the oil in a large skillet over medium heat.

4.   Divide the hash mixture into two (2) patties on the pan.

5.   Flatten them out a bit by pressing with a spatula.

6.   Cook each side for about 3 minutes or until golden brown.

7.   Serve with a slice of crispy bacon.

#3   Good Morning Sandwich

Ingredients:

2 egg whites

1 tbsp shredded cheese of your choice

1 tbsp chopped vegetable of your choice (e.g., carrot, green onion, spinach)

1 tbsp grilled turkey or chicken breast, chopped

Salt and pepper to taste

1 whole-wheat English muffin

Directions:

1.   In a microwave-safe bowl, mix together all the ingredients apart from the English muffin. Microwave this mixture on high for 1 minute.

2.   Take out and turn the egg mixture over and microwave for another 30 seconds to 1 minute.

3.   In the meantime, slice and toast the English muffin.

4.   Place the cooked egg mixture on the toasted English muffin.

#4   Beef, Spinach & Cheese Cups

Ingredients:

1 lb. ground beef

1 tbsp. thyme, chopped

2 cloves garlic, minced

1/2 tsp. paprika

1/2 tsp. ground cumin

1 1/2 cup spinach, chopped

½ cup white cheddar, shredded

12 quail eggs (if quail eggs are not available, use 12 small eggs)

1 tbsp. chives, chopped

Salt and pepper to taste

Directions:

1.   Preheat oven to 180°C.

2.   Lightly grease a muffin tin with cooking spray.

3.   In a mixing bowl, mix together the ground beef with thyme, garlic, paprika, cumin, salt, and pepper.

4.   Divide the mixture over the muffin tin. Press the mixture so that it goes up the sides to create a cup.

5.   Divide the spinach and cheese evenly over the cups.

6.   Crack an egg over the top of each cup.

7.   Bake for about 25 minutes, or until the eggs are set and the beef mixture is cooked through.

8.   Sprinkle the chives over the top just before serving.

#5   Cinnamon Overnight Oats

Ingredients:

50 grams steel-cut oats

1 tbsp chia seeds

1 tbsp dried dates, chopped

1 tbsp raisins

¼ tsp cinnamon

¼ tsp vanilla extract

160 ml almond or soy milk

80 g Greek yogurt, natural (unflavored)

Directions:

1.   Get a clean jar (or any container) that will fit all the above ingredients.

2.   Put all the ingredients in the order indicated above.

3.   Cover and put in the fridge overnight.

4.   Stir the next day and enjoy! (Note: if it's too dry for you, you can add a little more almond or soy milk.)

#6   Hearty Scrambled Eggs

Ingredients:

4 eggs, medium

1 tbsp grass-fed butter

2 cups spinach, chopped

1 clove garlic, minced

salt and pepper to taste

Directions:

1.   Heat a pan on medium-high heat and melt the grass-fed butter.

2.   In the meantime, crack and eggs in a bowl, add salt and pepper to taste, and then slightly scramble with a fork. Set aside.

3.   Put the garlic in the pan and lightly sauté until softened.

4.   Add the spinach and cook until just softened.

5.   Add the eggs and scramble with a spatula or wooden spoon.

6.   Remove the eggs from the heat. Optional: top with cheese and/or fresh herbs.

#7   Blueberry Pancakes

Ingredients:

1 cup whole-wheat flour

1 tsp baking powder

1/2 tsp baking soda

1/8 tsp salt

1 egg, lightly beaten

1 cup low-fat buttermilk

2 tbsp maple syrup alternatives: honey, agave sugar, coconut sugar)

Directions:

1.   In a bowl, whisk together the whole-wheat flour, baking powder, baking soda, and salt.

2.   In a separate bowl, mix together the egg, buttermilk, and maple syrup.

3.   Push the dry ingredients to the side to create a well in the center.

4.   Put the egg and buttermilk mixture in this space.

5.   Heat a nonstick pan to medium-high heat. Smear some butter on the pan and then drop 1/4 cupful of the batter on the pan.

6.   Cook until the edges begin to dry and bubbles appear at the top.

7.   Flip and cook for a few minutes more.

Lunch Recipes

For your sugar-free, low carbohydrate mid-day meals, you want something that will boost your energy for the remainder of the day, without making you feel too full. Otherwise, your sugar levels will skyrocket and you'll start to feel an 'energy slump' by mid-afternoon.

So here are seven (7) lunch recipes that will give you just the right amount of energy and nourishment.

#1   Beef Taco Avocados

Ingredients:

4 avocados

1 lime

1 tbsp. EVOO (extra-virgin olive oil)

1 onion, small, chopped

1 lb. ground pork

1 packet low-sodium taco seasoning

Salt and pepper to taste

Toppings:

1 cup shredded cheese

1/2 cup shredded lettuce

Greek yogurt (alternative: cottage cheese)

Directions:

1.   Cut the avocados in half and remove the pit.

2.   Scoop out some of the avocado, creating a bigger 'cup' to hold the other ingredients.

3.   Chop the avocado you removed. Squeeze a bit of lime juice over them so that they don't discolor. Set aside.

4.   Heat a pan or skillet over medium heat. Add (or spray) some EVOO.

5.   Add the onion to the pan and cook until softened.

6.   Add the ground beef and low-sodium taco seasoning. Season with salt and pepper, and cook the meat for about 6-7 minutes.

7.   Remove from heat and drain the fat.

8.   Fill each avocado half with the taco beef mixture.

9.   Top each mixture with the remaining cut avocado, cheese, lettuce, and Greek yogurt.

#2   Buffalo Shrimp Lettuce Wraps

Ingredients:

1/4 tbsp. butter

2 garlic cloves, minced

1/4 cup hot sauce

1 tbsp. EVOO (extra-virgin olive oil)

1 lb. shrimp, peeled and deveined

Salt and pepper to taste

1 head iceberg lettuce, leaves separated and washed (for serving)

1/4 red onion, finely chopped

1 rib celery, sliced thin

1/2 cup blue cheese, crumbled

Directions:

Buffalo sauce:

1.   Melt the butter in a saucepan over medium heat.
2.   Add the garlic and cook until fragrant.
3.   Add the hot sauce to the garlic butter and stir
4.   Turn the heat to low.

Shrimp sauté:

1.   In a separate skillet or pan, heat some oil over medium heat.
2.   Add the shrimp to the pan and season with salt and pepper.
3.   Cook the shrimps until they turn pink and opaque.
4.   Turn off the heat and add the Buffalo sauce to the shrimp mixture in the skillet. Toss to coat the shrimp.

Assembly:

1.   Get an iceberg lettuce leaf. Add a scoop of shrimp, and then top with red onion, celery, and blue cheese.

#3   Yummy Cauliflower Salad

Ingredients:

1 medium-sized cauliflower, cut into florets

6 slices bacon

1/2 cup Greek yogurt

1/4 cup full-fat mayonnaise

1 tbsp. lemon juice

1/2 tsp. garlic powder

1 1/2 cup cheddar, shredded

1/4 cup chives, chopped

Directions:

1.   Boil some water and then add the cauliflower florets.
2.   Steam the cauliflower for about 4 minutes, or just until fork-tender.
3.   Drain the cauliflower and set it aside to cool.
4.   Heat a non-stick pan over medium heat. Add the bacon and cook until crispy.
5.   Transfer the bacon to a paper towel-lined plate to drain excess fat. Once cool to handle, roughly chop the bacon.
6.   Mix together the Greek yogurt, mayonnaise, lemon juice, and garlic powder in a bowl.
7.   Add the steamed cauliflower and toss gently. Season with salt and pepper.
8.   Add in the bacon, cheddar, and chives.

#4   Tuna and Zucchini Cakes

Ingredients:

1 can tuna

1 medium zucchini

1 medium white onion, shredded (or sliced very thinly)

1 small carrot, finely chopped

Salt and pepper to taste

¼ tsp smoked paprika

2 large eggs, lightly beaten

1 tbsp whole wheat bread crumbs

Butter for frying

Directions:

1.   Open the tuna can and drain to get rid of excess liquid. Set aside.

2.   Shred the zucchini. Squeeze out as much excess liquid as you can.

3.   In a bowl, add the tuna, zucchini, white onion, carrot, salt and pepper, paprika, and lightly beaten eggs. Mix gently to combine.

4.   Shape the mixture into 1/2-inch thick patties

5.   Coat each patty in bread crumbs.

6.   Heat a non-stick pan over medium-high heat. Add some butter.

7.   Once the butter is melted, add the patties in batches so that they don't overcrowd the pan.

8.   Cook about 3-5 minutes on each side or until golden brown and the zucchini is cooked through.

#5   Pizza!

Ingredients:

1 whole-wheat pita

1/2 cup low-sodium tomato sauce

1/4 cup shredded mozzarella

1/2 cup grilled chicken or turkey breast

1/4 cup chopped sun-dried tomatoes

Garlic and oregano to taste

Salt and pepper to taste

Directions:

1.   Lightly toast the whole wheat pita bread.

2.   Take the pita bread out and top with 1 tbsp of tomato sauce.

3.   Add the rest of the toppings.

4.   Sprinkle with garlic and oregano,

5.   Place the pita back in the oven, put on 'broil' or 'grill' if possible, until the cheese bubbles.

#6   Spicy Tomato Soup

Ingredients:
1 tbsp butter
1 small white onion, chopped

2 cloves garlic, minced
1 tsp smoked paprika
4 medium tomatoes, chopped
1 cup chicken broth
1/2 cup cream cheese
salt and pepper to taste
fresh basil, optional for topping

Directions:
1.   Place a saucepan over medium-high heat. Melt the butter.
2.   Add the onion and garlic, and cook until fragrant and the onion is translucent.
3.   Add the tomatoes to the saucepan. Cook just until the tomatoes are soft.
4.   Add the chicken broth or stock to the pot and season with salt and pepper to taste.
5.   Bring everything to a simmer, and then lower the heat to medium-low. Simmer the soup for about 10 minutes.
6.   Turn off the heat.
7.   Puree the soup using a stick or immersion blender until your desired consistency.
8.   Optional: if you like your soup fine and without any 'bits', you can pass the soup through a fine sieve.
9.   Add the cream cheese to the soup and stir to dissolve.
10.   Ladle the soup into bowls, and garnish with lightly chopped fresh basil.

#7   It's A Wrap!

Ingredients:
2 large eggs
1/2 teaspoon hot sauce
Salt and pepper to taste
1 tbsp scallions, chopped
1 tbsp parsley, chopped

2 tbsp black bean dip

1 9-inch whole-wheat tortilla wrap

1 tsp extra-virgin olive oil

2 tbsp cheddar cheese, shredded

1 tbsp green or red salsa (optional)

Directions:

1.   Set your oven to 'broil'.

2.   Mix the eggs, hot sauce, salt and pepper, scallions, and parsley.

3.   If the black bean dip is cold, warm it up first in the microwave for a few seconds.

4.   Place the tortilla wrap between paper towels and warm in the microwave for a few seconds.

5.   Spread the warmed black bean dip over the wrap.

6.   Heat up a non-stick pan and brush some oil over it.

7.   Add the egg mixture and cook through.

8.   Place the skillet under the broiler and broil just until the top of the egg mixture is set.

9.   Slide the omelet on top of the wrap. Sprinkle with cheddar cheese.

10.   Roll the wrap and serve with salsa on the side (if using).

Dinner Recipes

Like many people, you probably look forward to a good dinner as a great way to end the day. Unfortunately, this is also why many tend to overeat at night. It's seen as a 'reward' after a tiring day.

Hopefully, after you try the breakfast and lunch recipes above, you'll soon discover that you don't head to dinner feeling starved and lacking energy. In fact, you might even feel the opposite and find yourself not wanting to eat as much as you used to during dinner time. Don't be surprised by this!

The recipes in this Healthy Eating for Healthy Living eBook are all designed to give you the RIGHT amount of energy throughout the day. No erratic energy highs and lows that lead to cravings, hunger pangs, and bingeing. So, let's get dinner cooking!

#1   Delish Mac & Cheese

Ingredients:

2 heads cauliflower, medium-sized, cut into florets

2 tbsp butter

1 cup heavy cream

150 grams cream cheese

4 cups cheddar, shredded

2 cups mozzarella, shredded

Salt and pepper to taste

Topping:

100 grams pork rinds, crushed

1/4 cup freshly grated Parmesan

1 tbsp extra-virgin olive oil

2 tbsp parsley, chopped for garnish

Directions:

1.   Preheat the oven to 190°C.

2.   Spray a 9x13-inch baking dish with cooking spray (or lightly butter it). Set aside.

3.   In a big bowl, add the cauliflower florets and two tablespoons of oil. Season with salt and pepper and toss.

4.   Spread the cauliflower onto two baking sheets. Roast them for about 40 minutes.

5.   While waiting for the cauliflower, warm the cream cheese in a big saucepan over medium heat.

6.   Once the cream cheese simmers, lower the heat to low.

7.   Add the cheddar and mozzarella cheeses. Stir until just melted, and then turn off the heat.

8.   Add the hot sauce and season the cheese mixture with salt and pepper.

9.   Add the roasted cauliflower and toss gently.

10.   Move the cauliflower and cheese mixture onto the prepared baking dish.

11.   Combine the pork rinds, parmesan, and oil in a medium bowl, and sprinkle this on top of the cauliflower and cheese mixture.

12.   Bake for about 15 minutes, or until the top becomes crusty and golden.

13.   Take out and garnish with parsley.

#2   Southern 'Fried' Chicken

Ingredients:

4-5 bone-in, skin-on chicken thighs (about 1 kilo)

salt and pepper to taste

2 large eggs

1/2 cup heavy cream

3/4 cup almond flour

1 1/2 cup pork rinds, crushed

1/2 cup Parmesan, grated

1 tsp. garlic powder

1/2 tsp smoked paprika

1/2 cup mayonnaise

1 1/2 tsp hot sauce

Directions:

1.   Preheat oven to 200°C.

2.   Place parchment paper n a big baking sheet.

3.   Pat the chicken thighs dry using paper towels and then season with salt and pepper.

4.   Whisk the eggs and heavy cream together in a bowl.

5.   In another bowl, mix together the almond flour, pork rinds, parmesan, garlic powder, and smoked paprika. Season with salt and pepper.

6.   Dip the chicken pieces one at a time into the egg mixture, and then into the almond flour mixture.

7.   Press the chicken pieces a bit into the almond flour to ensure they're properly coated. Place each coated chicken piece on the baking sheet.

8.   Bake for about 45 minutes, or until the chicken register an internal temperature of 74°C.

9.   Meanwhile, mix together the mayonnaise and hot sauce in a small bowl. Serve on the side with the 'fried' chicken.

#3   Miso Noodles With Chicken

Ingredients:

3/4 lb boneless, skinless chicken thighs

1 tbsp extra-virgin olive oil

1   bag   of   Japanese   buckwheat   soba   noodles

1/4 cup Shiro miso paste

1 tbsp low-sodium soy sauce

2 cups chicken or vegetable broth

5 stalks spring onions, sliced

1 tbsp sesame seeds, roasted

Directions:

1.   Thinly slice the chicken thighs. Season with salt and pepper.

2.   Put a non-stick pan on medium-low heat. Add the oil.

3.   Sauté the chicken pieces until cooked. Set aside.

4.   Cook the Japanese buckwheat soba noodles according to package directions. Set aside.

5.   In a saucepan, put the Shiro miso paste, soy sauce, chicken or vegetable broth, and spring onions to a gentle simmer.

6.   In a serving bowl, put the cooked chicken and drained soba noodles. Toss everything to combine.

7.   Ladle the miso soup over the bowls.

8.   Top with sliced spring onions and the roasted sesame seeds.

#4   Veggie Chili

Ingredients:

1 tbsp extra-virgin olive oil
1 small onion, chopped
3 cloves garlic, finely chopped

1 small green bell pepper, chopped
1 small red bell pepper, chopped
3/4 cup celery, chopped
3/4 cup dry red wine (or water)
2 cans diced tomatoes, undrained
1/4 cup tomato paste
2 cups vegetable stock
1 tbsp fresh cilantro, chopped
1 tbsp chili powder
1/2 tsp cumin
2 cans kidney beans, rinsed and drained

Directions:

1.   Heat a large pan over medium-high heat. Add the butter.

2.   Add the onion and garlic and cook until translucent.

3.   Stir in the green and red bell peppers, and celery.

4.   Add the wine and bring everything to a simmer.

5.   Add the tomatoes (with juice), tomato paste, vegetable stock, cilantro, chili powder, and cumin. Stir.

6.   Add in the kidney beans. Bring to a boil.

7.   Reduce the heat to low, cover, and cook, stirring occasionally, for about 45 minutes.

#5   Steak w/Salsa Sauce

Ingredients:

2 4-ounce, 1/2-inch-thick steaks (e.g., rib-eye)
1 tsp chili powder

Salt and pepper to taste

1 tsp extra-virgin olive oil

2 large tomatoes, diced

2 tsp lime juice

1 tbsp fresh cilantro, chopped

Directions:

1.   Trim the fat off the steaks.

2.   Rub both sides of the steak with chili powder, and salt and pepper.

3.   Heat the oil in a medium skillet (or grill pan) over medium-high heat.

4.   Add the steaks and grill, turning once until it the met reaches your preferred level of doneness.

5.   Put the steaks on a plate and cover them with foil. Let it rest while you make prepare the salsa.

6.   Using the same skillet, add the tomatoes, lime juice, salt, and pepper.

7.   Cook until the tomatoes soften.

8.   In a bowl, put together the tomato salsa, cilantro, and, if you like, the juices from the steak.

9.   Serve the steaks with the salsa on top.

#6   Mushroom and Scallion Chicken

Ingredients:

1 cup brown rice, cooked

100 grams shiitake mushrooms

250 grams boneless, skinless chicken thighs

salt and pepper to taste

1 tbsp sesame oil

1 garlic clove, finely chopped

2 cups water

2 tbsp cup low-sodium soy sauce

1 2-inch piece ginger, thinly sliced

3 stalks spring onions, sliced

Directions:

1.   Remove the stems from the shiitake mushrooms. Slice the mushroom caps thinly and set them aside.

2.   Slice the chicken thighs thinly. Season with salt and pepper. Set aside.

3.   In a big pot, heat the sesame oil over medium-low heat.

4.   Add the garlic and cook until fragrant.

5.   Add the shiitake mushrooms and cook until softened.

6.   Pour the water into the pot, and then add the soy sauce and ginger. Bring to a simmer. (Alternatively, you can use low-sodium chicken or vegetable broth. However, if you do this, reduce or completely omit the amount of soy sauce.)

7.   Add the chicken into the broth. Reduce the heat to low, cover, and then let the chicken poach until it's just cooked through.

8.   Divide the cooked brown rice over two bowls.

9.   Divide the chicken over the bowls. Pour the broth over the chicken, and garnish with spring onions.

#7   Sunday Meatballs

Ingredients:

1 lb ground beef

1 clove garlic, minced

1/2 cup mozzarella, shredded

1/4 cup Parmesan, grated

2 tbsp. parsley, chopped

1 large egg, beaten

Salt and pepper to taste

2 tbsp extra-virgin olive oil

1 medium onion, chopped

2 cloves garlic, minced

1 can crushed tomatoes

1 tsp dried oregano

Directions:

1.   In a big bowl, mix together the beef, garlic, mozzarella, parmesan, parsley, egg, salt, and pepper.

2.   Form about 15-16 meatballs from the mixture. Place the meatballs in the refrigerator for about 30 mins. (This will help keep its shape while cooking.)

3.   Heat the oil in a skillet over medium-high heat.

4.   Add the meatballs to the skillet, turning occasionally, and cook for around 10 minutes

5.   Remove the cooked meatballs and place them on a plate.

6.   In the same skillet, put the garlic and onion and cook until the latter is soft and translucent.

7.   Put in the tomatoes and oregano.

8.   Put back the meatballs. Season with salt and pepper, cover, and simmer for 12-15 minutes or just until the sauce has thickened.

Dessert & Snack Ideas

Just because you're on a sugar-free, low carbohydrate diet doesn't mean you should deprive yourself of yummy snacks and desserts! Try the following treats and be surprised at how satisfying they can be.

#2

Ingredients:

2 cups of Greek yogurt, unsweetened and unflavored

1 cup strawberries, frozen

1 cup mixed berries, frozen

1 tsp vanilla extract

1 tbsp honey or maple syrup

Directions:

1.   Put all the ingredients in a food processor, and process everything until creamy.

2.   Serve the ice cream immediately or put it in an airtight container and freeze until ready to serve.

#3   Mocha Chia Pudding

Ingredients:

1 tbsp chia seeds

1 tbsp cornstarch

2 tsp instant coffee mix (or espresso powder)

1/2 tsp ground cinnamon

1/4 tsp salt

1/4 cup raw honey (or maple syrup)

2 cups low-fat chocolate milk

50 grams dark chocolate (at least 70%), finely chopped

1 tsp vanilla extract

Directions:

1.   In a saucepan, mix together the chia seeds, cornstarch, coffee, cinnamon, and salt.

2.   Over medium heat, add the raw honey and chocolate milk. Stir and cook for 5 minutes, stirring often until the mixture thickens.

3.   Remove the mixture from the heat.

4.   Add the dark chocolate and vanilla, whisking fast to prevent lumps.

5.   Serve immediately. (Alternatively, you can put the mixture in a glass bowl. Cover it with plastic wrap directly on the surface and refrigerate for up to 5 days.)

#4   Banana Quesadillas

Ingredients:

1 whole wheat tortilla

1 large, very ripe banana

1 tbsp peanut butter

dark chocolate shavings (at least 70%, optional)

Directions:

1.   Mash the banana in a bowl with a fork.

2.   Get a tortilla wrap and spread peanut butter and the mashed banana on it.

3.   Add dark chocolate shavings.

4.   Fold or roll the tortilla.

5.   Warm in the microwave for about 20 seconds. Slice and serve.

#5   Mango & Coconut Treat

Ingredients:

1 mango, cut into wedges

1 tbsp dry, shredded coconut

Directions:

1.   Turn your oven to 'broil' and then position a rack in the upper third part of the oven.

2.   Line a baking tray with foil or parchment paper.

3.   Spread the dry, shredded coconut on a plate.

4.   Dip each mango slice into the shredded coconut, pressing each to fully cover.

5.   Arrange the mango slices in a single layer in the prepared pan and broil until the shredded coconut is nicely brown and slightly crispy.

#6   Sesame & Raisin Bombs

Ingredients:

1/3 cup honey (or maple syrup)

1/3 cup peanut butter

3/4 cup nonfat dry milk

3/4 cup sesame seeds

1/4 cup raisins

1/4 cup shredded coconut

Directions:

1.   Place the shredded coconut on a plate. Set aside.

2.   In a large bowl, thoroughly mix together the rest of the above ingredients.

3.   Using a small ice cream scooper (or a 1 tbsp measuring spoon), scoop out some mixture and roll into balls using your hands.

4.   Dip each ball into the shredded coconut.

5.   Place in the refrigerator for at least 4 hours before enjoying them.

#7   No-Bake Chocolate Cookie

Ingredients:

1.5 cups raw almonds

1.5 cups dates, un-pitted

1/4 cup cacao powder

1/2 tsp pure vanilla extract

1/4 tsp sea salt

Filling:

8 oz almond milk cream cheese

5 tbsp maple syrup

1/2 tsp pure vanilla extract

Directions:

1.   For the cookies: combine all the cookie ingredients into a food processor, and then process until everything comes together.

2.   For the filling: Set up your stand mixer using the paddle attachment. Add all the filling ingredients and whip until very smooth.

3.   Roll out the cookie 'dough' between two pieces of parchment paper until it's about 1/4 inch thick.

4.   Using a round cookie cutter, cut out cookie rounds and put them on a wide platter (or cookie sheet)

5.   Place the cookies in the refrigerator and chill for at least 30 minutes.

6.   Take the chilled cookies out.

7.   Place a half spoonful of cream cheese filling on one cookie and then top this off with another cookie round.

8.   Press slightly so that the cream cheese filling spreads out evenly inside the cookie.

9.   Eat right away or store the no-bake cookies in an airtight container in the refrigerator. They can last up to 7 days.

#8   Grapefruit Mango Sorbet

Ingredients:

1/4 cup water

2 tbsp cup cane sugar or coconut sugar

1/4 tsp ground ginger

1 large grapefruit, cut into segments

2 small scoops of mango sorbet

fresh mint (optional)

Directions:

1.   In a small saucepan, simmer the water, cane sugar, and ginger for about 5 minutes or until the mixture is reduced to a thick syrup.

2.   Divide the grapefruit segments over two dessert bowls.

3.   Pour the ginger syrup over grapefruit and top with each with a scoop of mango sorbet and fresh mint.

#9   Coconut Ice Cream

Ingredients:

2 cans thick, full-fat coconut milk

2 cup heavy cream

1/4 cup coconut sugar

1 tsp. pure vanilla extract

Pinch kosher salt

Directions:

1.   Chill the coconut milk in the refrigerator overnight.

2.   Open the coconut milk cans, and then spoon out the solidified coconut cream at the top. Using a hand mixer, whip the coconut cream until creamy. Set aside.

3.   In another bowl, using the hand mixer again, whip the heavy cream until soft peaks form.

4.   Add in the rest of the coconut milk, coconut sugar, and vanilla.

5.   Fold in the whipped coconut cream.

6.   Transfer the mixture into a loaf pan and freeze overnight.

#10   Healthy Popcorn

Ingredients:

2 tbsp coconut oil

1/2 cup popcorn kernels, unsweetened and unbuttered

Directions:

1.   Put a heavy-bottomed pot or pan over medium heat.

2.   Add the coconut oil and wait until it's melted.

3.   Take the pot off the heat. Add the popcorn kernels, cover the pot, and give it a quick shake to distribute the popcorn kernels inside it.

4.   Set the pot back on the stove burner and wait for the tell-tale popping sounds. Shake the pot every now and then to ensure that the heat is reaching all the kernels.

5.   Continue cooking until the popping sounds slow down to just about one pop per few seconds.

6.   Take off the lid and place the popcorn in a big bowl. You can sprinkle the popcorn with a bit of salt or smoked paprika.

#11   Veggie Platter with Homemade Hummus

Ingredients:

1 cucumber

1 carrot

3 celery stalks

1 red bell pepper

1 green bell pepper

1 cup cauliflower florets

For the hummus:

1 can chickpeas, drained but reserve the liquid

1/4 cup tahini

1 tbsp lemon juice

1 tbsp extra-virgin olive oil

1 clove garlic, grated

1/4 tsp ground cumin

Salt and pepper to taste

Directions:

1.   Slice all the vegetables, except the cauliflower, into sticks or whichever way you like them. (Note: Feel free to add any other vegetable you like too such as cherry tomatoes, olives, radishes, etc.) Arrange the vegetables on a big platter.

2.   To make the hummus, put all the ingredients in a food processor and blend until you reach your desired consistency. Adjust the seasoning if necessary.

3.   If the dip is too thick, add some water (or the drained chickpea water) a tablespoon at a time.

Bonus Recipes!

#1   Cauliflower Rice

Ingredients:

1 medium head cauliflower, cut into florets

1/2 tbsp garlic powder

1/2 tbsp turmeric powder

Salt and pepper to taste

Directions:

1.   Heat the oven to 200°C.

2.   Put the cauliflower florets into a food processor and 'pulse' until the cauliflower resembles rice granules.

3.   Spread the cauliflower rice onto a large baking tray.

4.   Add the garlic powder, turmeric powder, salt, and pepper. Mix to combine.

5.   Bake the cauliflower rice for 20-25 mins, mixing halfway through.

#2   REAL Chicken Nuggets

Ingredients:

4 pieces, boneless, skinless chicken thighs

1 cup buttermilk

1/2 tbsp garlic powder

1/2 tbsp onion powder

1/2 tbsp dried thyme

Salt and pepper to taste

1 egg

1 cup whole-wheat breadcrumbs

1/2 cup dried shredded coconut

Directions:

1.   Cut the chicken thighs into nugget-size pieces.

2.   In a bowl, mix together the buttermilk and half of the garlic powder, onion powder, and dried thyme.

3.   Place the chicken in the buttermilk mixture and refrigerate for at least 30 minutes. (Overnight is better.)

4.   Preheat the oven to 180°C.

5.   Lightly spray a baking sheet with cooking spray.

6.   Take the chicken out and drain from the buttermilk marinade.

7.   Lightly toast the whole wheat bread crumbs and shredded coconut.

8.   Place the bread crumbs and coconut on a shallow plate to cool. Once cooled, add the remainder of your seasonings to the plate.

9.   In a separate small bowl, lightly beat the egg.

10.   Dip each nugget into the egg mixture, then onto the breadcrumb mixture. Press to thoroughly coat the chicken.

11.   Place the nugget on the baking tray and do the same for all chicken pieces.

12.   Bake for about 10 minutes.

13.   Flip each nugget and bake for another 5 minutes or until the internal temperature of the chicken reaches 74°C.

#3   Baked Sweet Potato Wedges

Ingredients:

2 medium sweet potatoes

1/2 cup extra-virgin olive oil

Salt and pepper to taste

2 tbsp rosemary, finely chopped

Directions:

1.   Preheat the oven to 200°C.

2.   Wash and brush the sweet potatoes to get rid of any dirt.

3.   Slice the sweet potatoes into wedges, and then place them in a shallow bowl.

4.   Add the extra-virgin olive oil, rosemary, salt, and pepper. Toss to combine.

5.   Place the wedges on a baking sheet and bake for 30-35 minutes.

#4   Avocado Chips

Ingredients:

1 large ripe avocado

1/2 cup Parmesan, grated

1 tsp lemon juice

1/2 tsp garlic powder

1/4 tsp dried oregano

Salt and pepper to taste

Directions:

1.   Preheat the oven to 175°C.

2.   Lightly spray two large baking sheets with cooking spray or line them with parchment paper.

3.   In a bowl, mash the avocado with a fork.

4.   Add the grated Parmesan, lemon juice, garlic powder, dried oregano, salt, and pepper to the avocado mash.

5.   Using a small ice cream scooper or a measuring spoon, scoop out a tablespoon of the mixture to the baking sheet. Leave space around each scoop, about 3 inches.

6.   Using the back of a wet spoon, spread and flatten the mixture thinly.

7.   Bake the 'chips' for around 30 minutes, or until crisp and golden.

8.   Cool and serve.

#5   Whole Wheat Banana Loaf

Ingredients:

1/3 cup coconut oil, melted

1/2 cup raw honey (or maple syrup)

2 large eggs

1/4 cup water, filtered

2 large very ripe bananas

1 tsp vanilla extract

1/4 tsp salt

1/2 tsp cinnamon

1.5 cups whole wheat flour

1 tsp baking soda

Directions:

1.   Preheat the oven to 165°C.

2.   Lightly grease a 9×5 inch loaf pan.

3.   In a big bowl, whisk together the coconut oil and raw honey. Add the eggs and water. Mix well to combine.

4.   Peel and mash the bananas.

5.   In a separate bowl, mix together the bananas, vanilla, salt, and cinnamon.

6.   Add the banana mixture to the wet ingredients. Stir to combine.

7.   Whisk the whole wheat flour and baking soda together. Add this to the rest of the ingredients. Stir just to combine.

8.   Place the batter into the greased loaf pan.

9.   Bake for 55-65 minutes. To test if the banana loaf is done, insert a toothpick in the middle of the bread and take it out after a few seconds. If it comes out clean (i.e., hardly any crumbs are attached to it), the bread is done.

10.   Cool the banana loaf for about 5 minutes. Remove from the loaf pan and move to a wire rack to cool for another half hour before slicing and serving.

Zero Sugar, Low-Carb Friendly Drinks

Apart from water, is there anything else you can drink? Yes, plenty! Following are some options for you. Of course, it goes without saying that the following drinks should be consumed as is, which means no adding of any sugar or sweetener whatsoever.

1.   Herbal tea.

Open yourself to the widely varied world of tea! Tea flavors range from light floral blends to deep and warm earthy flavors so there's a wide assortment to choose from. You can have it hot or cold too. Best of all, tea contains no sugar!

Tea also offers A LOT of health benefits depending on the ingredient you use. For instance, chamomile tea is known to heal sinus issues and even migraines. Mint tea improves digestion and oral health. Ginger tea is great against sore throats and is known to boost the body's immune system. Rooibos tea, an herbal tea from South Africa, is believed to help with weight loss.

Healthy example: Natural Chamomile Flower Tea

Boil about a liter of water in a kettle or water boiler. Pinch off about 3-4 tablespoons worth of chamomile flowers direct from its stems. Put the boiled water into a teapot and let the chamomile flowers infuse in it for about 5 minutes. Drink and enjoy. (You can add a sprig of peppermint or a whole cinnamon stick in the pot too as well.)

2.   Lemon- or lime-infused water.

Who says you should only have this at fancy restaurants? Get yourself a nice, tall glass pitcher, fill it with filtered water and add a whole lemon or lime (or both!) cut into thin slices. Sip this hydrating, sugar-free drink throughout the day and see your skin improve too.

3.   Fruit- or herb-infused water.

There's no need to confine yourself to citrus fruits. Flavor your water with fruit and/or herbs as well. The only thing with this option is that they may need some time. You can pretty much drink brewed teas and lemon/lime water immediately. Fruit and herbs, however, need a few hours to steep before they can really impart their flavors to the water.

Healthy example: Watermelon and Mint Water

Cut up some watermelon into chunks and put them in a pitcher. (Alternatively, you can use an infusion water bottle for on-the-go drinking.) Get some mint leaves and bruise them using the back of a knife. Add the mint to the watermelon and top it all off with filtered water. Set this in the fridge to cool for 4-5 hours.

4.   Flavored or unflavored sparkling water.

Many people trying to quit sugar find it extremely hard to switch to plain water because of their HIGH consumption of soda drinks. The answer to that is sparkling water. Start with the flavored variety like peach mango, strawberry, cranberry, etc., and then gradually graduate to plain carbonated water. Before you know it, you'll be ready to switch to plain water in no time.

5.   Coffee!

Skip the 1,000 calorie Frappuccino and go back to basics – have plain, unadulterated black coffee. Drip it, cold brew it, ice it, French press it. It doesn't matter. The rule of thumb is to have coffee as 'pure' as possible.

If you can't bear to switch to 'plain black' just yet, then add cinnamon or nutmeg to your cup. Just not sugar! You may also want to try changing coffee brands or testing other coffee flavors.

As your eating lifestyle changes, so will your taste buds. So don't be surprised that you find your coffee tasting 'different' now. It may not be just the lack of sugar.

I would of course suggest that you stick to just plain water or any of the zero sugar alternatives above from here on out. But if you do find yourself wanting just a tiny bit of sugary taste in your drinks, then I recommend the following.

6.   Freshly-squeezed lemonade.

Lemonade brings memories of lazy summer days and sticky fingers. Bring back the fun without the added sugar by making a simple syrup from healthy sweetener options like cane sugar, coconut sugar, raw honey, or agave nectar.

Boil a cup of water on the stove, and then add a cup of your healthy sweetener of choice. Stir to dissolve the sweetener and then remove the syrup from the heat. Juice a cup of lemon juice into a pitcher. Add 3 cups of filtered water and then add HALF of the simple syrup. Serve chilled with ice and fresh lemon slices.

7.   Coconut water.

Did you know that coconut water has low sugar content? With just 8-10 grams of sugar per cup, it's a great and refreshing alternative to water. It has many health benefits too.

Coconut water may lower blood sugar levels, help prevent the formation of kidney stones, has antioxidant properties, and is a great source of calcium and potassium.

8.   Kombucha.

Kombucha has been making waves in the health and wellness niche. And while its slightly sweet, slightly sour flavor is not for everyone, it's believed to have probiotic qualities which are great for gut health.

9.   Plant-based milk.

Cow's milk is not recommended while on a zero sugar diet because it contains natural sugar. Of course, that's still better than ADDED SUGAR but why not try plant-based milk instead such as almond milk, macadamia nut milk, or even flaxseed milk. Of course, go for the unsweetened versions of these milk alternatives.

Can you JUICE on a zero sugar diet?

It really depends on the *juice ingredients*. When people think of 'juicing', it's all about fruits. That's not good if you're on a zero sugar diet because fruits are high in natural sugars. What you should do, if you really want to juice, is to juice a healthy mix of fruits AND vegetables. Here are some juicing recipes you can try.

The Salad Juice

1 head romaine lettuce

1 handful of spinach

1 celery stalk

3 kale leaves

1 lemon, peeled

1-inch knob of fresh ginger

The 'Hulk'

1/2 green apple

3 kale leaves

8 mints

3 limes, peeled

1 cucumber

1 handful of spinach

Blackberry Green Juice

1/2 cup fresh blackberries

1/2 green apple

1 lemon, peeled

3 kale leaves

1/2 cup broccoli

1/2 cup fresh watercress

1/2 small cucumber

The Gut Health Juice

1 fennel stalk

1 celery stalk

1-inch knob of fresh ginger

1 big carrot

3 kale leaves

1/2 small cucumber

1 lemon, peeled

Beet It

1 small red beet

1 small carrot

1-inch knob of fresh ginger

1 lemon, peeled

2 handfuls spinach

1 celery stalk

The directions for the above juice options are the same: wash the ingredients thoroughly. If applicable, peel the produce. Put all the ingredients through a juicer and enjoy!

Note that it's best to drink fresh juice within 24 hours. Anything longer and the juice will start to lose some of its nutritional benefits.

Chapter 8
Improve Your Health Inside and Out

There's no doubt about it. Adapting a zero sugar, low carbohydrate eating lifestyle will do WONDERS for your health. And as you start your healthy living journey, I do recommend that you stick to making dietary changes first.

You see, the reason many people fail with their weight loss and/or healthy living efforts is that they take on too many things too soon.

So I say – focus on healthy eating first.

Once you see the amazing results that healthy eating brings, go ahead and take further steps regarding your health and fitness levels.

Trust me – you WILL want to do more than just eat healthy once you start losing weight and feeling more energetic.

But once you reach that stage, what do you do? That moment is the perfect time to address your **mental health** and **physical fitness** levels.

Mental - Mindset Changes Toward Food

Life throws A LOT of curveballs. You know this. You're bound to encounter certain life events (e.g., birthday parties, Holiday dinners, work-related celebrations, etc.) that may make you stumble with your healthy eating, healthy living habits.

And that's OK!

Here are a few mindset changes you may need to adapt to help you positively move on if ever you go 'off track'.

1.   Food is NOT your enemy.

Here's the truth – food was never your enemy. In the beginning, your *food choices* may have been your undoing. However, as we discussed in Chapter 2, sugar is addictive. So, in many ways, you were compelled to make unhealthy food choices later on.

So here's the mindset change you need to adapt – stop thinking of unhealthy food as the enemy you need to defeat.

In fact, go ahead and enjoy unhealthy foods **once in a while**, and **in moderation**.

2. Food is not a measure of yourself as a human being. Food does not define you. Many people undergoing dietary changes feel that if they slip and eat unhealthy food, they somehow fail as a person. This is not a healthy mindset to have.

Food is there to nourish your body; to give you the right energy so that you can live life to the fullest. It should not define you as a person.

Instead, I suggest you list down all your GOOD qualities. If you lost your way while you were leading an unhealthy life, it's time to get to know yourself again!

Listing down your positive qualities will not only boost your mood but will also remind you that you're MORE than your food choices.

Often, when someone is asked to write down what they like or what's good about themselves they don't want to do it because they think it's being vain. Not at all! It's ALWAYS better to be positive than to be negative about yourself.

Another obstacle is that people often don't know WHAT to list down about themselves. Well, let me help you.

Following are a few questions I encourage you to answer now.

- What do you like about yourself?
- What positive characteristics do you have?
- What are some of your achievements?
- What are some challenges (big or small) that you've overcome?
- What talents or skills do you have?

Are you still finding it hard to say something great about yourself? Here's another question.

What has a friend done for you lately?
Sample answer: She cooked and sent me some soup when I was not feeling well.

Now, ask yourself this: would I do something like that for a friend who's sick?

If you say yes, then you can list down the following positive qualities for yourself.

- I am a great friend.
- I have empathy.
- I'm someone people can count on.

3. Think and consider before you eat something.

Every time you're faced with an unhealthy food item, take a few seconds and ask yourself – *is this worth it?*

If it's not, let it go and move on to a healthier alternative.
If it is, go ahead and enjoy it.
If it's not and you eat it anyway, enjoy it, and then get back on track tomorrow.

That's it. Move on.

The point is that you shouldn't dwell on it. Contemplating it over and over simply makes it a big issue in your mind when in reality it isn't or it doesn't have to be!

4. Willpower has nothing to do with your zero sugar journey.

Willpower is the ability to fight short-term temptation in favor of long-term goals. But instead of trying to practice 'willpower' every single day, why not just make a slight modification in your mindset and character?

For example, why not say "I will only eat chips on weekends; Saturday or Sunday night only."

All of a sudden you removed any feelings of deprivation and instead made a decision to eat chips only on weekends. The *pressure* of trying to avoid chips Monday to Friday is gone because you've delegated the decision to the weekend.

Try it now. Close your eyes, take a deep breath, and think of ONE trigger food with which you struggle. Open your eyes, let your breath out, and state your rules.

Examples:
- I will eat one slice of chocolate cake, but only during birthday parties. (So if there's no chocolate cake at the next birthday party you attend, no cake for you.)
- I will drink one alcoholic beverage during parties, but only if I'm with Tina. (So if Tina's not with you, you don't drink alcohol.)

5. Let go of shame.

    Did you know that shame can be a negative, and paralyzing emotion?[38]

    Ok, so you indulged in some deep-fried chicken, pasta carbonara, a slice of cake, and a few glasses of wine last night.

    Many people on a health or weight loss journey would wake up feeling ashamed by this. But it's not the food that may prove to be your undoing. It's the feeling of shame that you associate with it.

    Shame can be a self-defeating emotion that if you give in to it – you may end up giving up what you've accomplished altogether. (This is the 'if I can't stick to my plan, then I better give up' mentality)

    So here's the mindset shift you need to make – accept that you gave in, take responsibility for it, and then get back directly on your healthy lifestyle routine.

6. Healthy eating is SELF-LOVE.

    Many people think that switching to a healthier eating pattern is all about deprivation. That it's a punishment to eat healthily. They're wrong.

    Healthy eating is practicing self-care and self-love.

    Do you want to age gracefully? Do you want to look older, or younger than your real age? Do you want to be out of breath all the time and have difficulty moving, or do you want to be flexible and energetic now and in the years to come?

Do you see it? Choosing to eat healthy means you love yourself because you want to live a long and happy life.

7. Keep moving forward.

You're losing weight and feeling great – good for you! Don't stop now. Keep moving forward!

Learn and educate yourself more about food, your body, and what you like and dislike about health and well-being in general.

For instance, many people on a zero sugar, low carbohydrate diet find themselves learning about a new world of ingredients. So perhaps now would be a good time to travel and deepen your knowledge about a specific food ingredient (e.g., travel to India to know about different spices).

Don't want to travel? Then how about just taking an online course about meal prepping, or cooking more vegetarian dishes?

Truly, the world is your oyster.

Physical - Move Your Way to Fitness

One of the ways to move forward and build on your healthy eating, healthy living success is to **GET PHYSICAL.** Yes, we're talking about movement, being more physically active, exercising!

If you want to lose weight and be healthier, then yes, changing your eating lifestyle is enough to melt the pounds. However, if you want to tone your body and improve your fitness levels, then you need to move.

Besides, what are you going to do with all the EXTRA ENERGY you have after following my 7-Day Zero-Sugar Diet Plan?

And in case you're still on the edge about WHY you should exercise, let the following facts persuade you.

1. Exercise FIGHTS sickness and diseases. Physical activity improves your body's high-density lipoprotein (HDL) cholesterol levels while lowering unhealthy triglycerides in your body. This health combo drastically lowers your risk of contracting cardiovascular illnesses.

   Consistent exercise helps prevent many health issues such as stroke, metabolic syndrome, high blood pressure, type 2 diabetes, different types of cancer, arthritis, and others.

Exercise also boosts cognitive function, improving memory and thinking functions.

2. Exercise improves your mood. Exercise releases *endorphins*, chemicals that relate with receptors in your brain to lower pain perception. It also stimulates chemicals that can make you feel happier, less stressed, and more relaxed. So if you ever need an emotional lift, get moving!

Regular exercise also improves your physical appearance, which in turn can boost your self-confidence and self-esteem.

3. Exercise gives you even more energy. Regular exercise improves muscle strength and advances your physical endurance. This is because physical activity delivers oxygen and nutrients to body tissues and helps your cardiovascular system work better. As a result, you'll have more energy to do daily tasks and chores.

4. Exercise supports quality sleep. Yes, you'll feel tired after an exercise session but in a GOOD way. As such, it can help you sleep faster and experience better quality sleep. However, don't exercise strenuously just before bedtime as this may leave you too energized to sleep. If you want to use exercise for the purpose of winding down, then a light, meditative yoga session is ideal.

5. Exercise boosts 'bedroom activity'. If you lack energy and have a negative body image of yourself as a result of being overweight, it's understandable that intimacy in the bedroom takes a backseat.

The good news is that with consistent exercise, you can increase energy levels and your self-confidence, which in turn can revive your sex life.

But it's not just about having more energy. Exercise itself enhances arousal in women because it increases and sustains levels of an enzyme that boosts genital blood flow and arousal.

6. Exercise supports long-term, permanent weight loss.[39] Regular exercise helps maintain weight loss and prevent future weight gain. This is because exercise helps the body burn calories. The more strenuous the exercise routine, the more calories are burned.

However, note that you DO NOT need a fancy gym membership to establish an effective exercise routine.

No equipment workouts: take the stairs instead of the elevator at work, run outdoors, engage in bodyweight exercises, dance, and more!

When possible, invest in inexpensive equipment like a pair of dumbbells, a gym ball, elastic bands, or even a hula hoop!

Do remember though that **consistency is key**. Keep moving to keep burning calories.

7.   Exercise can open a whole new social network for you! Believe it or not, exercising can lead to new friends. For example, early morning walks or jogs can reveal others in your neighborhood who have the same routine. Start with a smile, nod, or wave as a greeting. Next time, strike up a short and easy conversation. Who knows where that will lead?

If you're attending local exercise classes at your local gym, great! You already have a group of people interested in the same thing as you are. Again, don't be afraid to start a short and easy conversation with someone. Everything starts with 'hello'.

So, how much physical activity do you need?
According to the U.S. Department of Health and Human Services, adults should engage in a combination of aerobic and strength activities each week.[40]

Aerobic exercises are any activities that promote cardiovascular conditioning. Anything that requires a bit of effort and gets your heart rate up will do.

Following is what's recommended for aerobic activities.

  ➢   Do at least 2.5 hours of light to moderate aerobic activity, or 75 minutes of energetic aerobic activity each week. A combination of light and dynamic aerobic activity is ok too.
  ➢   Spread out your exercise times over the week. That is, it's better for your heart and your overall condition to do 30 minutes of aerobic activity per day than exercising for 2 full hours on a weekend.
  ➢   For greater health benefits and to assist with weight loss success and maintenance, a minimum of 300 minutes (1 hour a day, 5 days) is recommended.

Strength training, also known as weight training or resistance training, builds muscle endurance and thus makes your body stronger.

Following is what's recommended for strength training.

- ➤ Perform strength training exercises targeting all major muscle groups at least twice a week.
- ➤ Try to perform at least one set of every strength training exercise using a resistance level that's hard enough to tire your muscles. (One step is equivalent to about 12-15 repetitions.)

Sample 14-Day Fitness Routine for Beginners

If you're new to fitness activities, that's ok! No one expects you to burst out the front door, and participate in a half marathon. Slow but sure is the key. Remember, **everyone starts at Level 1.**

The outline below is a simple fitness guide for beginners. Try and do the aerobic exercise for at least 30 minutes each day. If you can't do that, start at 15 minutes each day and work your way up.

Notice that the strength training exercises are not introduced until the following week. If you feel fit and have the time to incorporate them on Day 1, great! If not, that's ok too.

What's important is this – START!

Day	Aerobic Exercise	Strength Training Exercise
Day 1	Brisk walking*	
Day 2	Power walking**	
Day 3	Brisk walking	
Day 4	Power walking	
Day 5	Brisk walking	
Day 6	Power walking	
Day 7	Brisk walking + Light jog***	

D ay 8	Brisk walking + Light jog	Bodyweight squats[a]
D ay 9	Power walking + Light jog***	Beginner plank[b]
D ay 10	Power walking + Light jog	Bodyweight squats
D ay 11	Brisk walking	Beginner plank
D ay 12	Power walking	Bodyweight squats
D ay 13	Brisk walking + Light jog****	Beginner plank
D ay 14	Light jog	Full plank

<u>Fitness Notes:</u>

* **Brisk walking** – just walk a little bit faster than your CURRENT walking speed. The goal is simply to be a little bit out of breath, but nothing that you cannot manage for 15-30 minutes straight.

** **Power walking** –walk a little bit faster than your brisk walking pace. Add some PROPER arm swinging if you can. How? Bend your elbows at 90 degrees. Don't clench your hands, relax them. Keep your elbows close to your body, and let them naturally swing back and forth as you walk.

*** **Brisk/Power walking + Light jog** – Brisk walk or power walk, and then light jog at intervals. For example, brisk walk for 10 minutes, and then lightly jog for 1 minute. When this gets easy, brisk walk for 10 minutes and then lightly jog for 3 minutes. Keep on going and increasing the light jogging minutes as your aerobic endurance improves.

The end goal is to be able to lightly jog for 15 or 30 minutes straight.

Other light aerobic exercise ideas: swimming, biking, cycling, dancing, etc.
As for strength training exercises, I suggest you do them immediately after your aerobic exercises. Your muscles are all warmed up at this stage, so it's best to do them now.

If time does not permit that, then make sure you do some warm-up exercises for at least 5 minutes before squatting or planking.

[a] **Bodyweight squats** are one of the easiest resistance exercises you can do. Simply stand straight with your feet hip-width apart. Tighten your stomach muscles, and then start lowering yourself down as if you're going to sit on a chair. Pause and then stand back up. Repeat the movement until you do 12-15 repetitions.

[b] **Beginner planks** are not only easy to do anytime, anywhere; they also target A LOT of muscles in the body so it's a great weight training activity.

The image below is for a full plank, which is the goal

For a beginner plank, bring your knees to the floor and extend your arms (i.e., don't bend your elbow). Hold the pose for 5 seconds. If you can do it longer, great! If not just build upon that time, going from 5 seconds to 10 seconds, to 15 seconds, and so on.

Once you hit 60 seconds, move on to do a full plank and build the time you can hold that pose until you reach 60 seconds.

From there, you can do dozens of plank variations such as side planks, plank jacks, up and down planks, side tap planks, body saw planks, and much more.

Other beginner strength training exercise ideas: walking lunges, bear crawl, dumbbell rows, etc.

Leave a 1-click review!

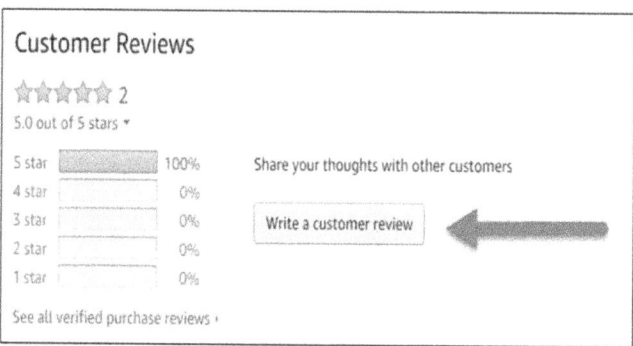

I would be incredibly grateful if you take just 60 seconds to write just a brief review on Amazon, even if it's just a few sentences.

https://www.amazon.com/review/create-review-asin=B09MCXR9T5

Conclusion

I t's great you decided to prioritize and take care of yourself and I thank you for selecting the Healthy Eating for Healthy Living guide as your health journey partner.

Author Thomas Sterner said **"Everything in life worth achieving requires practice"**, and that is definitely true for anyone embarking on a zero sugar, low carbohydrate eating lifestyle.

Your attempts at kicking sugar and its harmful effects on your life may be tough and frustrating at times but I assure you – if you follow what I outlined in this eBook, and keep on practicing these strategies, **YOU WILL SUCCEED.**

I know because as I mentioned at the start, I was just like you.

I was feeling miserable, not liking the way I was looking, letting myself and people around me down, and worst of all, **I was truly starting to believe that I couldn't change anything – UNTIL I DID.**

Today, I got up bursting with energy and excited about the day ahead. I look forward to what I need to do, knowing that I'm more than physically able to do them.

I'm mentally and emotionally stable and love the woman I see looking right back at me in the mirror.

And it all starts with KNOWLEDGE.

In this eBook, you learned that:
- ➢ Sweet, sugary foods are not feel-good friends. They're health adversaries that diminish the quality of life.
- ➢ Sugar addiction is REAL. However, just like any learned compulsion, you can unlearn it!
- ➢ Adapting a zero sugar, low carbohydrate eating lifestyle gives you benefits **beyond weight loss. You increase your body's ability to heal from** sugar-related illnesses; you boost your energy levels; you sleep better; you improve your gut health; you lower your risk of contracting life-threatening diseases such as cancer; you improve brain function; you improve your emotional and mental state. And so much more!

➤ Success depends on the right preparation. To triumph with a zero sugar diet plan, it's important to set yourself up for success by doing things like clearing out your kitchen of unhealthy food items, learning mindful eating techniques, discovering non-food-related rewards, educating yourself on how to shop for healthy food, and so on.

➤ Living a healthy life is NOT about deprivation; it's about proper substitution.

➤ Meal planning and meal prepping can mean the difference between a healthy meal and an unhealthy one.

➤ Avoiding sugar is more than just paying attention to what you eat and drink. Your MIND plays a vital role in healing your sugar addiction.

And of course, thanks to the easy recipes in Chapter 7, you learned that healthy eating is not so difficult a change after all.

Truly, everything you need to lead a happier, healthier, and longer life is here. There's only one thing left to do - START.

Note: If you found this eBook useful, do not forget to leave a review on Amazon to let others know how much you appreciated it. Thank you very much!

My other books you will love!

Amazon.com/dp/B09MJ5282Q

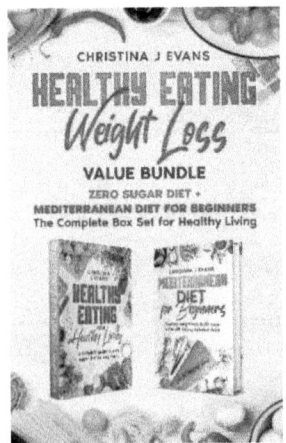

Amazon.com/dp/B09MHF2XQ1

Don't forget to grab your GIFT!!!

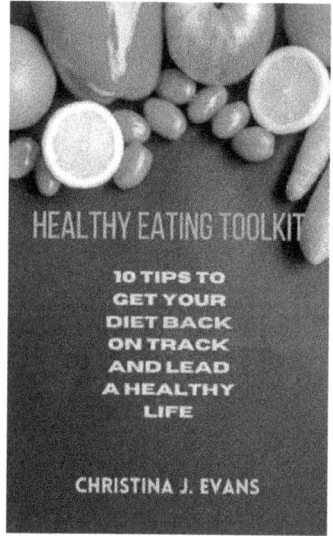

http://christinajevans.com/healthy-eating.pdf

Joining the HL Community

Looking to build your healthy eating lifestyle? If so, then check out the Healthy Living (HL) Community here:

www.facebook.com/groups/1004091000384321/

Appendices

Appendix A – A List of Grocery Staples and their Glycemic Load

A low glycemic load (GL) value keeps blood sugar levels consistent so that you don't experience that roller-coaster style of sugar highs and crashes. And since it's very important to regulate blood sugar levels for effective weight loss, the table below shows GL levels. As a general rule, the lower the GL value the better it is for a zero sugar, low carbohydrate diet.

ITEM	GLYCEMIC LOAD	SERVING SIZE
Vegetables		
Broccoli, cooked	0	78g (1/2 cup)
Cabbage, cooked	0	75g (1/2 cup)
Celery, raw	0	62g (1 stalk)
Cauliflower	0	100g (1 cup)
Green Beans	0	135g (1 cup)
Mushrooms	0	70g (1 cup)
Spinach	0	30g (1 cup)
Carrot, raw	1	15g (1 large)
Tomato	1.5	123g (1 med)
Peas, Frozen	3.4	72g (1/2 cup)
Beets, canned	9.6	246g (1/2 cup)
Parsnip	11.6	78g (1/2 cup)
Sweet Potato	12.4	133g (1 cup)
Yam	16.8	136g (1 cup)
Fruits		
Avocado	0	50g
Lime	1	120g
Strawberry	1	120g
Apricot	3	120g
Grapefruit	3	120g
Lemon	3	120g

Cantaloupe	4	120g
Guava	4	120g
Nectarines	4	120g
Oranges	4	120g
Pear	4	120g
Watermelon	4	120g
Blueberries	5	120g
Peach	5	120g
Plum	5	120g
Apple	6	120g
Pineapple	6	120g
Kiwi	7	120g
Mango	8	120g
Cherries	9	120g
Prunes	10	60g
Banana	11	120g
Grapes	11	120g
Oats		
Steel-cut oats		
Old-fashioned or whole oats		
Quick or instant oats (unflavored)		
Nuts (Raw, Unsalted/Unroasted)		
Almonds	0	30g (handful)
Walnuts	0	30g (handful)
Pistachios	0	30g (handful)
Peanuts	0	30g (handful)
Cashew	0	30g (handful)
Fats & Oils		
Extra Virgin Olive Oil		
Coconut oil		
Grass-fed butter		
Pasta, Breads, Rice		

Pasta/Bread: anything as long as they're whole-wheat or whole grain		
Rice: brown rice		
Canned Goods		
Canned tuna		
Canned salmon		
Meat/Protein		
Chicken	Eggs	
Beef	Lamb	
Fish	Pork	
Bacon (Go for the 'center cut'. The leaner the meat, the better.)		

Appendix B – The Most Common Sugar Names

One of the reasons it's so difficult to eliminate sugar from our diets is because they go by so many names! Following is a list of the most common sugar names today. Note that not all of the sugars listed below are bad per se. It's the amount of sugar that counts. As a rule of thumb, a total carbohydrate count of is 1–2 grams is still ok to consume in a low carbohydrate eating lifestyle.

Basic Simple Sugars (monosaccharides and disaccharides):	
1.	Dextrose
2.	Fructose
3.	Galactose
4.	Glucose
5.	Lactose
6.	Maltose
7.	Sucrose
Solid or Granulated Sugars:	
8.	Beet sugar

9.	Brown sugar
10.	Cane juice crystals
11.	Cane sugar
12.	Castor sugar
13.	Coconut sugar
14.	Confectioner's sugar (aka, powdered sugar)
15.	
16.	Corn syrup solids
17.	Crystalline fructose
18.	Date sugar
19.	Demerara sugar
20.	Dextrin
21.	Diastatic malt
22.	Ethyl maltol
23.	Florida crystals
24.	Golden sugar
25.	Glucose syrup solids
26.	Grape sugar
27.	Icing sugar
28.	Maltodextrin
29.	Muscovado sugar
30.	Panela sugar

31.	Raw sugar
32.	Sugar (granulated or table)
33.	Sucanat
34.	Turbinado sugar
35.	Yellow sugar
	Liquid or Syrup Sugars:
36.	Agave Nectar/Syrup
37.	Barley malt
38.	Blackstrap molasses
39.	Brown rice syrup
40.	Buttered sugar/buttercream
41.	Caramel
42.	Carob syrup
43.	Corn syrup
44.	Evaporated cane juice
45.	Fruit juice
46.	Fruit juice concentrate
47.	Golden syrup
48.	High-Fructose Corn Syrup (HFCS)
49.	Honey
50.	Invert sugar
51.	Malt syrup

52.	Maple syrup
53.	Molasses
54.	Rice syrup
55.	Refiner's syrup
56.	Sorghum syrup
57.	Treacle

References

1. Centers for Disease Control and Prevention. (2021, September 27). *Heart disease facts*. Centers for Disease Control and Prevention. Retrieved October 1, 2021, from https://www.cdc.gov/heartdisease/facts.htm.

2. *2019 Philips World Sleep Day Survey Results - United States*. (n.d.). Retrieved October 1, 2021, from https://www.usa.philips.com/c-dam/b2c/master/experience/smartsleep/world-sleep-day/2019/2019-philips-world-sleep-day-survey-results.pdf.

3. Spiegel, K., Tasali, E., Penev, P., & Cauter, E. V. (2004). Brief communication: Sleep curtailment in healthy young men is associated with decreased leptin levels, elevated ghrelin levels, and increased hunger and appetite. *Annals of Internal Medicine, 141*(11), 846. https://doi.org/10.7326/0003-4819-141-11-200412070-00008

4. Breymeyer, K. L., Lampe, J. W., McGregor, B. A., & Neuhouser, M. L. (2016). Subjective mood and energy levels of healthy weight and overweight/obese healthy adults on high-and low-glycemic-load experimental diets. *Appetite, 107*, 253–259. https://doi.org/10.1016/j.appet.2016.08.008

5. Lim, S. Y., Kim, E. J., Kim, A., Lee, H. J., Choi, H. J., & Yang, S. J. (2016). Nutritional factors affecting mental health. *Clinical Nutrition Research, 5*(3), 143. https://doi.org/10.7762/cnr.2016.5.3.143

6. McClain, A. D., van den Bos, W., Matheson, D., Desai, M., McClure, S. M., & Robinson, T. N. (2013). Visual illusions and plate design: The effects of plate rim widths and rim coloring on perceived food portion size. *International Journal of Obesity, 38*(5), 657–662. https://doi.org/10.1038/ijo.2013.169

7. Hitti, M. (2008, July 8). *Weight loss study: Keeping a food diary helps shed extra pounds*. WebMD. Retrieved September 1, 2021, from https://www.webmd.com/diet/news/20080708/keeping-food-diary-helps-lose-weight.

8. Johnson, R. K., Appel, L. J., Brands, M., Howard, B. V., Lefevre, M., Lustig, R. H., Sacks, F., Steffen, L. M., & Wylie-Rosett, J. (2009). Dietary sugars intake and cardiovascular health. *Circulation, 120*(11), 1011–1020. https://doi.org/10.1161/circulationaha.109.192627

9. Avena, N. M., Rada, P., & Hoebel, B. G. (2008). Evidence for sugar addiction: Behavioral and neurochemical effects of intermittent, excessive sugar intake. *Neuroscience & Biobehavioral Reviews, 32*(1), 20–39. https://doi.org/10.1016/j.neubiorev.2007.04.019

10. Faruque, S., Tong, J., Lacmanovic, V., Agbonghae, C., Minaya, D., & Czaja, K. (2019). The dose makes the poison: Sugar and obesity in the United States – A Review. *Polish Journal of Food and Nutrition Sciences, 69*(3), 219–233. https://doi.org/10.31883/pjfns/110735

11. Delli Bovi AP;Di Michele L;Laino G;Vajro P; (n.d.). *Obesity and obesity related diseases, sugar consumption and bad oral health: A fatal epidemic mixtures: The pediatric and odontologist point of View.* Translational medicine @ UniSa. Retrieved October 1, 2021, from https://pubmed.ncbi.nlm.nih.gov/28775964/.

12. R, O., B, G., & KR, U. (n.d.). *low carbohydrate Diet.* Europe PMC. Retrieved September 1, 2021, from https://europepmc.org/article/NBK/nbk537084.

13. Quagliani, D., & Felt-Gunderson, P. (2016). Closing America's fiber intake gap. *American Journal of Lifestyle Medicine, 11*(1), 80–85. https://doi.org/10.1177/1559827615588079

14. Harvey, C. J., Schofield, G. M., & Williden, M. (2018). The use of nutritional supplements to induce ketosis and reduce symptoms associated with keto-induction: A narrative review. *PeerJ, 6.* https://doi.org/10.7717/peerj.4488

15. B;, A. K. A.-S. E. A.-S. (n.d.). *The effect of tongue scraper on mutans streptococci and lactobacilli in patients with caries and periodontal disease.* Odonto-stomatologie tropicale = Tropical dental journal. Retrieved September 1, 2021, from https://pubmed.ncbi.nlm.nih.gov/16032940/.

16. *The link between taste buds, obesity, more.* Cornell Research. (2019, November 7). Retrieved September 2021, from https://research.cornell.edu/news-features/link-between-taste-buds-obesity-more.

17. *Losing weight, especially in the belly, improves sleep quality, according to a Johns Hopkins Study - 11/06/2012.* Johns Hopkins Medicine, based in Baltimore, Maryland. (n.d.). Retrieved September 2021, from https://www.hopkinsmedicine.org/news/media/releases/losing_weight_especially_in_the_belly_improves_sleep_quality_according_to_a_johns_hopkins_study.

18. Rejeski, W. J., Ip, E. H., Bertoni, A. G., Bray, G. A., Evans, G., Gregg, E. W., & Zhang, Q. (2012). Lifestyle change and mobility in obese adults with type 2 diabetes. *New England Journal of Medicine, 366*(13), 1209–1217. https://doi.org/10.1056/nejmoa1110294

19. *Dealing With Feelings When You're Overweight.* Rady Children's Hospital-San Diego. (2014, September). Retrieved September 1, 2021, from https://www.rchsd.org/health-articles/dealing-with-feelings-when-youre-overweight/.

20. Burri, B. J. (2011). Evaluating Sweet Potato as an intervention food to prevent vitamin A deficiency. *Comprehensive Reviews in Food Science and Food Safety, 10*(2), 118–130. https://doi.org/10.1111/j.1541-4337.2010.00146.x

21. Matito, C., Agell, N., Sanchez-Tena, S., Torres, J. L., & Cascante, M. (2011). Protective effect of structurally diverse grape procyanidin fractions against UV-induced cell damage and death. *Journal of Agricultural and Food Chemistry, 59*(9), 4489–4495. https://doi.org/10.1021/jf103692a

22. Fat and salt combined is a toxic mix for our health and waistlines. (2016, March 10). Retrieved from https://www.deakin.edu.au/about-deakin/news-and-media-

releases/articles/fat-and-salt-combined-is-a-toxic-mix-for-our-health-and-waistlines.

23. Fernstrom, J. D. (2007). Health issues relating to monosodium glutamate used in the Diet. *Reducing Salt in Foods*, 55–76. https://doi.org/10.1533/9781845693046.1.55

24. Kristeller, J. L., & Hallett, C. B. (1999). An exploratory study of a meditation-based intervention for binge eating disorder. *Journal of Health Psychology*, 4(3), 357–363. https://doi.org/10.1177/135910539900400305

25. About the Author: Chris Dunne Marketing Executive at Tameday., & Tameday., M. E. at. (2019, May 3). *Do naps at work increase productivity?* Tameday. Retrieved September 2021, from https://www.tameday.com/do-naps-at-work-increase-productivity/.

26. Mayo Foundation for Medical Education and Research. (2020, August 18). *Exercise and stress: Get moving to manage stress*. Mayo Clinic. Retrieved October 26, 2021, from https://www.mayoclinic.org/healthy-lifestyle/stress-management/in-depth/exercise-and-stress/art-20044469.

27. Stenblom, E.-L., Egecioglu, E., Landin-Olsson, M., & Erlanson-Albertsson, C. (2015). Consumption of thylakoid-rich spinach extract reduces hunger, increases satiety, and reduces cravings for palatable food in overweight women. *Appetite*, 91, 209–219. https://doi.org/10.1016/j.appet.2015.04.051

28. Belluz, J., & Zarracina, J. (2016, April 28). *Why you shouldn't exercise to lose weight, explained with 60+ studies*. Vox. Retrieved October 1, 2021, from https://www.vox.com/2016/4/28/11518804/weight-loss-exercise-myth-burn-calories.

29. Xu, A. J., Schwarz, N., & Wyer, R. S. (2015). Hunger promotes acquisition of nonfood objects. *Proceedings of the National Academy of Sciences*, 112(9), 2688–2692. https://doi.org/10.1073/pnas.1417712112

30. Wansink, B., Hanks, A. S., & Kaipainen, K. (2016). Slim by design. *Health Education & Behavior*, 43(5), 552–558. https://doi.org/10.1177/1090198115610571

31. Leidy, H. J., Clifton, P. M., Astrup, A., Wycherley, T. P., Westerterp-Plantenga, M. S., Luscombe-Marsh, N. D., Woods, S. C., & Mattes, R. D. (2015). The role of protein in weight loss and maintenance. *The American Journal of Clinical Nutrition*, 101(6). https://doi.org/10.3945/ajcn.114.084038

32. Westerterp, K. R. (2004). Diet induced thermogenesis. *Nutrition & Metabolism*, 1(1), 5. https://doi.org/10.1186/1743-7075-1-5

33. Dai, H., Milkman, K. L., & Riis, J. (2014). The fresh start effect: Temporal landmarks motivate aspirational behavior. *Management Science*, 60(10), 2563–2582. https://doi.org/10.1287/mnsc.2014.1901

34. Helander, E. E., Wansink, B., & Chieh, A. (2016). Weight gain over the holidays in three countries. *New England Journal of Medicine*, 375(12), 1200–1202. https://doi.org/10.1056/nejmc1602012

35. *Food Safety and Inspection Service*. Home | Food Safety and Inspection Service. (n.d.). Retrieved October 26, 2021, from https://www.fsis.usda.gov/.

36. Benedict, K., Jackson, B. R., Chiller, T., & Beer, K. D. (2018). Estimation of direct healthcare costs of fungal diseases in the United States. *Clinical Infectious Diseases, 68*(11), 1791–1797. https://doi.org/10.1093/cid/ciy776

37. Martins, N., Ferreira, I. C., Barros, L., Silva, S., & Henriques, M. (2014). Candidiasis: Predisposing factors, prevention, diagnosis and alternative treatment. *Mycopathologia, 177*(5-6), 223–240. https://doi.org/10.1007/s11046-014-9749-1

38. Sussex Publishers. (n.d.). *Overcoming the paralysis of toxic shame*. Psychology Today. Retrieved October 26, 2021, from https://www.psychologytoday.com/us/blog/overcoming-destructive-anger/201704/overcoming-the-paralysis-toxic-shame.

39. RIEBE, D., BLISSMER, B., GREENE, G., CALDWELL, M., RUGGIERO, L., STILLWELL, K., & NIGG, C. (2005). Long-term maintenance of exercise and healthy eating behaviors in overweight adults. *Preventive Medicine, 40*(6), 769–778. https://doi.org/10.1016/j.ypmed.2004.09.023

40. U.S. Department of Health and Human Services. (n.d.). Physical Activity Guidelines for Americans Summary - 2nd edition.

Lightning Source UK Ltd.
Milton Keynes UK
UKHW040639201221
395966UK00001B/105

9 781915 301000